THE THREE LOST BOOKS OF HEALING

SUE YOUNG

Spring 2001 – Autumn 2004

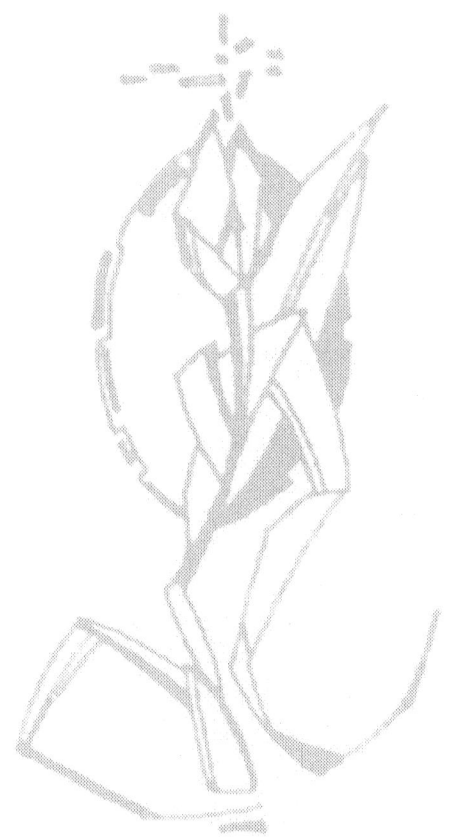

Second edition Winter 2005

Published by Sue Young
sue@wildfalcon.com
homeopathy.wildfalcon.com

ISBN 1-4116-6431-0

Printed by Lulu
313 RDU Centre Drive
Suite 210
Morrisville, North Carolina 27560
United States

Additional copies available at the above address or from www.lulu.com

Typeset in Gill Sans and ITC Galliard
Designed by Laurie Robert Young and Jessica Schilling

From a primal act of Nature when lightning strikes the Earth,
we can sense the original fusion.
Fire above meets the Earth below.
This wonder comes from outside ourselves, from the universe.
White ash, red Earth and black charcoal.

These three colours are our original colours.
Their source was our original wonder, our original trauma.
We learnt awe here.
We learnt to think here.
We learnt to paint here.

This is the origin of life and death.
This is the origin of kindness and cruelty, of love and hate.
This is the origin of trauma and of healing.
We watch as death claims life.
We watch as life grows out of the charred remains of death.
It is apparent that both states arise from each other.
It is apparent that both states are equal and opposite.
It is apparent that we are looking in a Mirror.

This secret truth is so simple we do not perceive it.
If we can understand this secret, we can sense our own origins,
we can understand the universe.

I have observed during my 50 years in this World, that this secret truth
is the essence of healing. Its simplicity has always kept it hidden. I was
taught that the best way to hide something is in plain sight, so I lay
before you the Three Lost Books of Healing. They are only fragments of
the Great Work, but they are the Key!

Sue Young

CONTENTS

THE LOST WHITE BOOK OF HEALING

Assault	2	Instinct	27
Balance	3	Introvert	28
Change	4	Invasion	29
Chaos	5	Kindness	30
Circle	6	Language	31
Collapse	7	Covert Language	32
Common Sense Procedures	8	Healing Language	33
Confusion	9	Official Language	34
Corkscrew	10	Subjective Language	35
Cruelty	11	Life	36
Death	12	Magnetic	37
Detoxification	13	Mirror	38
Disease	14	Motivation	39
Distortion	15	Physical Damage	40
Electric	16	Potential	41
Exhaustion	17	Prejudice	42
Extrovert	18	Process	43
Fate	19	Spiral	44
Fragmentation	20	Stereotype	45
Fusion	21	Survival	46
Gathering	22	Taboo	47
Growth	23	Trauma	48
Healing	24	White	49
Hope	25	Wisdom	50
Inappropriate Treatment	26		

THE LOST RED BOOK OF HEALING

Awareness	54	Joy	79
Balance	55	Justice	80
Change	56	Language of Power	81
Chaos	57	Language of Weakness	82
Circle	58	Life	83
Collapse	59	Love	84
Common Sense Procedures	60	Magnetic	85
Death	61	Manoeuvre	86
Direction	62	Mirror	87
Disease	63	Motivation	88
Distortion	64	Palate	89
Electric	65	Past	90
Enemy	66	Permission	91
Environment	67	Potential	92
Escape	68	Process	93
Evolve	69	Red	94
Fate	70	Spinning	95
Freedom	71	Spiral	96
Friend	72	Strength	97
Future	73	Survival	98
Growth	74	Trauma	99
Hate	75	Understand	100
Healing	76	Universe	101
Imprint	77	Wisdom	102
Inappropriate Treatment	78		

THE LOST BLACK BOOK OF HEALING

Awareness	106	Justice	131
Balance	107	Knowledge	132
Black	108	Language of Defeat	133
Circle	109	Language of Future	134
Common Sense Procedures	110	Language of Past	135
Confusion	111	Language of Wisdom	136
Contentment	112	Life	137
Dancing	113	Love	138
Death	114	Magnetic	139
Destiny	115	Mirror	140
Direction	116	Past	141
Disease	117	Permission	142
Distortion	118	Perpetrator	143
Electric	119	Potential	144
Enemy	120	Present	145
Environment	121	Process	146
Existence	122	Scapegoat	147
Fate	123	Singing	148
Fear	124	Spiral	149
Friend	125	Strength	150
Future	126	Truth	151
Hate	127	Understand	152
Healing	128	Universe	153
Hierarchy	129	Wisdom	154
Inappropriate Treatment	130		

" 'Such a storm of emotions as humans evoke, all on the basis of imagination', the dragon observed condescendingly. In a more reflective voice, she asked, 'Do you do this because you live such short lives? Tell yourselves wild tales of what might happen tomorrow, and feel all the feelings of events that will never happen? Perhaps to make up for the past you cannot recall, you invent futures that will not exist.' "

Robin Hobb
The Liveship Traders: The Ship of Destiny
HarperCollins 1999

THE LOST WHITE BOOK OF HEALING

To Giaan.

New Life.
"Life is the strongest force in the universe.
You live within the universe.
The universe lives within you.
The past is inside you.
The future is dedicated to you."

January 2002

In order to be fully alive, we need to gather together all that we are, heal ourselves, and then realise our potential.

Anything that prevents this process is disease.

ASSAULT

Any assault on life will cause trauma and distortion.
This will provoke a reaction from life.
It will trigger healing and survival, or collapse and death.
The circle turns endlessly!
Life becomes a stereotype, bent out of shape.
Thus, assault directs life by impacting upon it.
The spiral turns endlessly!

The corkscrew of imperfect thinking fans the flames.

Knowing the process makes healing easier.

"For the power of a man's mind when it is perverted and corrupted by love
of evil is so great that he gives assent neither to his own nor to other men's
judgement but prefers to go against his own conscience – and everyone
else's – rather than resist what he loves with such intense passion."

Pelagius on Riches
B R Rees Pelagius: Life and Letters
Boydell 1991

BALANCE

Such a cacophony of experience.
Such a complex maelstrom.
Spinning endlessly, circling, spiralling in a multitudinous assault.
How do we direct ourselves?
What do we need, what do we want, what will aid us,
what will damage us, what will feed us, what will save us?
How do we simply exist?

Laws determine structure.
The only constant is change.
There is a process occurring here.
If you are aware of the process you can steer yourself.
You can amuse yourself,
bouncing off walls or trying to avoid them until you get the idea.
Fate is just guesswork at this point!
If you are an immortal soul, this may take a while!
If not, then consider the footsteps you are leaving for others to follow.
Either way, fate will affect us all in the end.
Eventually, we all shut up and listen.

This is balance!

"After all the disillusionments with which the history of civilisations is studded
– the triumphs of savagery, the bloodlettings of barbarism, the reversals of
progress, the reconquests by Nature, our failing to improve – there is no
remedy except to go on trying and keeping civilised traditions alive."

Felipe Fernandez Armesto
Civilisations
Macmillan 2000

CHANGE

The only constant in the universe is change.
Nothing stays the same!
In health, life copes with change. It adapts and grows.
If this ability to react to change is damaged, trauma and disease occur.
Healing demands change.
We cannot stay in our damaged state,
where distortion and fragmentation are the rule.
We need to move and grow out of these uncomfortable states.
If we stay in disease, we could collapse and die.
Luckily, change often occurs as a result of disease,
which causes the process of healing to occur automatically.
Luckily, change often occurs as a result of life,
which causes the process of disease to occur automatically.
The circle turns, the spiral spins.
The stream of consciousness moves imperceptibly.
Wisdom will eventually occur, fate will see to that!
All else is death.

"What are you when sleeping?
A body or a spirit;
Or a being of light?
O skilful minstrel,
Will you not answer?
Know you where night
Awaits the day?
Know you how many leaves are on the bush?
How the mountain was raised
Before the elements settled?
What supports the World,
What makes it habitable ...?"

Taliesin
John Matthews
Aquarian 1991

CHAOS

Balancing chaos can be tiring!
Keep a grip!
Understand that chaos is chaos!

There are laws governing chaos, so what do we know about the rules?
The rule is there is no law!
Fate is just guesswork at this point!

If we have structures, we can orient ourselves and guide ourselves
as we negotiate through experience.
Chaos has no structure.
We have to find other strategies!

Knowing this makes survival possible.
It gives us a chance of success where none existed before.
Such an imperceptible change to the possibilities and probabilities
of such an encounter will be all we get!

We have done so much for so long with so little
that now we can do anything with nothing!

"It is fitting that this book should end with the mention of results
which point the way to a host of future developments, by no means the
least of which is the question of how to quantize a system
which is classically chaotic!"

T W B Kibble and F H Berkshire
Classical Mechanics, fourth edition
Chapter 14, 'Order and Chaos ...'
Longman

CIRCLE

To avoid distorted, corkscrew thinking, it is important
to gather all possible information into a circle of illumination.
Otherwise, you just have a stereotype, nothing more!

Every issue needs to be investigated from every angle, every dimension,
through time, through close contacts.
Every living being is in a constellation with others, we are all social beings.
From individual to culture, to society to species,
from future predictions to knowledge of origins, all must be considered.

We must try to perceive the structure of the whole.
Nothing can be left out.
Knowing this prevents distortion.

"In our contemporary world of instant everything, these three
exercises call us to remember the cyclical nature of life and personal
growth. Whether it takes the form of cleansing, setting things right in a
relationship or the completion of one of life's cycles, taking the time to
acknowledge and make conscious what you are about to do will invariably
enrich your experience."

R Blum
The Book of Viking Runes
Headline 1993

COLLAPSE

Sometimes, life dies.
Sometimes, it will suffer fragmentation and distortion.
Sometimes, it will shut down some parts to save other parts.

Each collapse is a mirror of the assault that caused it.
The reflection forms part of the dance of life and death.
Its forms are infinite.
Survival is not always the outcome.
Equations will be finely worked.

Thus, studying the original trauma
is crucial to understanding the reaction of life to it.

The circle turns, the spiral spins and fate intervenes.
The stream of consciousness continues.
Electric and magnetic charges flicker around the scene.

Wisdom and kindness dictate that common sense procedures
and detoxification will help to prevent physical damage,
and inappropriate treatment should be avoided.
Exhaustion must be addressed.

"The Capacity to become ill seems to be built into the ground plan of
human nature regardless of mental efforts to the contrary. Moreover, we
are not merely free floating minds, but minds embodied."

Edward Whitmont
Psyche and Substance
North Atlantic 1980

COMMON SENSE PROCEDURES

Find at least three people you can confide and communicate with
for support during the healing and recovery process.
This is called a three-legged stool.
Don't be afraid to extend this basic structure
to others who are prepared to help.
This releases you from the need to confide randomly
with inappropriate contacts and thus suffer social censure.
If you are not currently communicating with anyone, this is vital.
Engage effectively with your "three legged stool" support structure
and prepare for an honest assessment of your situation.
Learn to release massive build-up of trapped emotional wind safely.
Learn about the process.
Grasp the fact that healing is possible.
Avoid inappropriate treatment.
Avoid corkscrew thinking.
Do not use stereotypes.
Do this quickly!
Learn about detoxification, as there are commonly chemical,
bacteriological and toxicological underpinnings to trauma and disease.
Learn to take care of yourself and attend to your diet.
Don't try giving everything up at once, but learn to make gradual changes.
Exhaustion must be addressed.
Do everything you can to prevent physical damage.
Learn about kindness.
Do this very slowly!

"Overworked and exhausted. Sits and thinks about little affairs that
amount to nothing. Worries about all their responsibilities and duties.
Averse to work or exertion. Inability to apply himself. Learns poorly. Low
spirited. Apathetic. Depressed. Melancholic or doubting moods.
Hopeless of ever getting well."

Robin Murphy
Calcarea Carbonica, Homoeopathic Materia Medica
Lotus Star Academy 1995

CONFUSION

Fragmented pieces of arguments crash together into false logic.
Any stereotype spins the corkscrew of imperfect thinking,
which will cause chaos, given half a chance.
Prejudice and cruelty are the children of disease.

Complicated issues arouse many different points of view,
all competing together, all intruding into all discussions.
These issues need separating into piles in order to be clearly perceived.
They then need to be compared across piles,
reformed into different piles, sifted, recombined and sorted endlessly
into infinite combinations of infinite diversity.
Piles need to be understood in terms of interdependence,
independence, difference, similarity, contrast and identity.
Anything that prevents this process is disease.
Remember that all things combine to become whole.
Remember that all things have a tendency to separate
to make new combinations.

Confusion is consciousness changing.
It is growth, it is change and it can lead to wisdom.
Hope springs out of confusion.
Such a small imperceptible wisp is all we will get out of the maelstrom.
Is it enough?

"... who regards the mystics not only as the ultimate source of knowledge
of the soul and its capacities and defects,
but as the salt which preserves human societies from decay."

Aldous Huxley
The Perennial Philosophy
Chatto and Windus 1950

CORKSCREW

Limiting human thought to either/or choices is a sad option.
Human experience is vastly more complex.

Removing shadow from debate is uncomfortable.
Ideas need to wriggle around a bit and get comfortable.
The more information gathered, the subtly different any decision will be.

Language is very complex.
It has always been used to manipulate herds,
direct reality and promote world-views.
The less information gathered, the more successful the stereotype.
The more useful the spin!
Discrete choices are no more that sub-totals in the chain of thought,
and they impact on health directly.
Forcing an either/or decision on a complex system
eradicates multiple realities and can cause distortion and trauma,
even catastrophic reactions.
Discrete points in the stream of consciousness
are only aids to understanding.
Prejudice and cruelty feed voraciously on the killing ground
left by imperfect thinking of the corkscrew.
Circle around the spiral until you glimpse the dance.

"The person who loves crime lives in it. It becomes a part of his nature
and shows itself in the external man. The man who loves truth and
humanity, lives in that idea, and it becomes a part of his nature, and can
be seen in his looks and in his life."

J T Kent
Lesser Writings on Homeopathy
B Jain 1987

CRUELTY

The corkscrew perverts language and results in distortion and trauma,
ultimately leading to violence and disease.

Cruelty is a killing ground, but it requires prejudice to flourish.
Its tools are assault, invasion, trauma and taboo.

Such actions mirror the fragmentation of the perpetrator.
They cause similar magnetic and electric reactions from the scapegoat.

Both invoke fate.

Pain felt is pain given is pain received in an endless invasion of life.

This is disease.
This is violence.
Death is triumphant.

"Profound melancholy with tendency to use foul, violent language.
Malicious, seems bent on wickedness. Absence of all moral restraint.
Hard-hearted, cruel, fixed ideas."

Robin Murphy
Anacardium Orientale, Homoeopathic Materia Medica
Lotus Star Academy 1995

DEATH

Death is part of life.
We are all finite creatures.
Death is the only option if life cannot be maintained.
Each living being will assess the equation
of survival, motivation and disease.
The result will not always equal life.

We are also infinite creatures,
as our actions, words and deeds can go on influencing life after we die.
Mortal or immortal beings,
we spend our time half with life and half with death.
It is an endless dance.
The death of an old idea, an old way of being, an old mode of thinking,
a old basis of belief always leads to change and to growth.
This releases our potential.
As such, death is part of life.
Death is taboo to most, feared and avoided and misunderstood.
Prejudice and distortion lead to stereotypes, not wisdom.
Corkscrew thinking forms poor assessments and bad equations
as to our true nature.

So where is hope?

"Try not to turn away from those whose appearance is disturbing, from the ragged and unwell. Try never to think of them as inferior to yourself. If you can, try not even to think of yourself as better than the humblest beggar. You will all look the same in your grave."

The Dalai Lama
Ancient Wisdom, Modern World
Little, Brown and Co 1999

DETOXIFICATION

In health, life is self-repairing and self-cleaning
and can easily maintain itself over a lifetime.
If life is damaged through assault, invasion or trauma,
living beings can no longer operate effectively.
The inability of a system to clean itself is often the first detectable symptom.
This often goes unnoticed until it causes disease.

If life is blocked or clogged or entangled or distorted or damaged,
then secondary elimination routes take over.
The resultant sufferings are almost always diagnosed as
conditions in themselves and suppressed one way or the other.
Inappropriate treatment can lead to physical damage and death.

Life become stuck and disease proliferates.
Common sense procedures are advised.
Exhaustion must be addressed.
Detoxification is a continuous process.
One-off treatments can shock the system, so it is best done gently,
little and often and with kindness.
Bodies eliminate via the bowel, the kidneys and the skin and by breathing.
Psychological detoxification is more complex,
but basically, the process is the same.
No matter where the trauma originated,
it will all end up in the toilet eventually!

"Overactive mind. Nervous and excitable. Very irritable, sensitive to all
impressions. Cannot bear noises, odours, light. Angry and impatient,
cannot stand pain, so mad he cries. Zealous, fiery temperament. Aversion
to work. Fears poverty. Sullen. Spiteful. Nagging. Violent. Suicidal,
homicidal impulses. Fear of knives, lest she should kill herself or others."

Robin Murphy
Nux Vomica, Homoeopathic Materia Medica
Lotus Star Academy 1995

DISEASE

Disease is an assault on life.
This causes fragmentation and distortion of life.
It causes alteration and fluctuation in life.

In the body, this process is seen via symptoms.
In the emotions, disturbance can be observed.
In the mind, intellectual processes struggle.
In the spirit, abnormal states occur.

Disease is observable as a shock wave rippling out.
Then a secondary reaction from life can be detected.
All levels are disturbed.
This distortion can be obvious or subtle.

Disease takes many forms.
The reaction of life in response is equally complex.
Many complex continuums interact here.
Balance is the key.

Understanding this makes healing easier.

"The diseases to which man is liable are either rapid morbid processes of
the abnormally deranged vital force ... acute disease ...
or they are diseases of such a character that, with small, often
imperceptible beginnings, dynamically derange the living organism, each
in its own peculiar manner, and cause it gradually to deviate from the
healthy condition ... chronic disease.."

Samuel Hahnemann
Aphorism 72, The Organon of Medicine
B Jain

DISTORTION

Distorted functioning can quickly lead to disaster.
Subtle changes can be as devastating as major changes.

Distortion can be the first sign of change.
It can lead to growth.
Subtle changes can be as vital as major changes.
This is a dangerous time!

The corkscrew of imperfect thinking can lead to distortion
and fragmentation and possible collapse of living systems.
The proliferation of symptoms can lead to physical damage.
Emotional states become abnormal.
Spiritual processes become disturbed.
The confusion of imperfect thinking can lead to balance and healing
and possible change in living systems.
The proliferation of life can lead to gathering and kindness.
Emotional states normalise.
Spiritual thinking addresses fate.
Cruelty and prejudice are the children of disease.
Hope and wisdom are the children of our potential.

"Sickness is like a sitar whose correct tuning has been disturbed.
Naturally, all the notes from such a sitar will be far from melodious.
There is no use trying to correct the individual notes. It is the disturbance
in the tuning itself which has to be corrected."

Rajan Sankaran
The Spirit of Homoeopathy
Homoeopathic Medical Publishers Bombay 1994

ELECTRIC

Electricity is very sudden.
It is either there or it is not there.
Magnetic energy distorts in the aftermath.
Its very suddenness can cause trauma.
Its absence can reduce motivation and lead to death.
Like fire, it is a good servant, but a poor master.

The drama of this energy in living beings is grossly misunderstood.
Its effect on us is profound,
but obvious in ways that are of vital importance to our nature.
If we ignore it, we misunderstand ourselves utterly,
knowing what we miss.
If we embrace it, we are in danger of physical damage.

Balance is the key.

"Disease and death are the result of two active forces. One is the will of
the soul, which says to the instrument: I draw the essence back.
The other is the magnetic power of the planetary life, which says to the
life within the atomic structure: the hour of re-absorption has arrived.
Return to me. Thus, under cyclic law, do all forms act."

Alice Bailey
Esoteric Healing
Fort Orange 1978

EXHAUSTION

We all think we know what exhaustion is.
However, our definition may be simple over-exertion or over-working,
a short-term condition easily remedied by a good holiday
or a few days in bed!

The sort of exhaustion that builds up over months or years
as living beings battle trauma and disease
and distortion and fragmentation is rarely understood.
When healing reaches the stage when recovery is close,
the body gives up this hidden backlog.
It can take a long time to recover from this wall of exhaustion,
which now breaks like a dam.

This release and the resultant detoxification
will trigger regeneration of living beings
by demanding nourishment, rest, quietness and slow peaceful days.
Physical limits will be restricted by a healing body that can only give finite
amounts of energy in short bursts, to prevent physical damage.
It is time to pay the piper
for all those times spent operating well beyond our design specifications!

"Listless and dullness. Impaired memory. Brain fag. Apathetic.
Indifferent to everything. Settled despair. Aversion to talking.
Cannot collect his thoughts or find the right words.
Difficult comprehension. Effects of grief or mental shock.
Homesickness with inclination to weep. Delirium with great stupefaction.
Mild delirium, easily aroused. Hopelessness. Hysteria at change of life.
Dread of future, broods over one's condition."

Robin Murphy
Phosphoric Acid, Homoeopathic Materia Media
Lotus Star Academy 1995

EXTROVERT

Some of us like to extend and engage with others.
We like to vocalise and interact.
We like to discuss ideas and talk long on each issue.
We tend to take others' counsel above our own.

This strategy bruises others who have a different approach
and do not need others' counsel to make decisions.
They tend to become quieter and more withdrawn around extroverts,
as their usual practices are denied.

Each is offended by the other, even though we all use
many different strategies at different times and in different situations!

Knowing this prevents distortion and invasion.
Knowing this prevents prejudice.
Knowing this prevents corkscrew thinking.
Knowing this makes healing easier.

"One feels that homoeopathy is not clearly understood; it has been the
Cinderella of medicine for so long; it is time that this lowly handmaiden
should shed her cloak of humility and come out of her obscurity and
boldly proclaim what good she can do."

D Shepherd
The Magic of the Minimum Dose
Health Science Press 1985

FATE

Are we responsible for our actions?

Some people say our actions determine our fate,
a process intimately connected to the dance of life and death.

If reincarnation is true,
then we are immortal beings governed by our fate.
Some people think we are mortal beings
and our actions are not determined by fate, but they are legally binding
and have social implications that will eventually impinge on us.
What goes around, comes around!

Either way, our actions are intimately connected to our fate.
If we assume that we can act with impunity,
then we allow distortion and use corkscrew thinking,
which leads to taboo, prejudice, assault and invasion.

Whatever our beliefs, our actions will eventually affect us,
the society around us, and the social and political reactions
and the religious structures they evoke.

Knowing this promotes healing.

"We simply recognise that man himself, if observed in depth, and the
ultimate aim of his passage through the World, discloses an implicit
tendency to self-realisation in a determined direction."

Dr Proceso Sanchez Ortega
Notes on the Miasms

FRAGMENTATION

When distortion and disease reach critical levels, life becomes contorted.
In extremis, it will react.
Like a spring, it will snap back to grid.
Or it will break.
Or, it will do both at once!
This needs to be understood on all levels.
The body may need a remedy.
The emotions may need a reaction.
The mind may desire an answer.
The spirit may need an idea.
Or we will need all of them at once!
Taken together, disease and the reaction of life against it
are equal and opposite forces.
From the contorted pattern seen in the fragments,
footprints can be identified.
Magnetic distortion demonstrate these fragments were originally whole.
Electric discharge flickers around the fragments, keeping them apart,
but joining them together, demonstrating their origin.
All that can be seen is a stereotype.
Wisdom is hidden.
Hope is crying.

"Perfection calls imperfection to the surface. Good drives evil always from the form of man in time and space. The method used by the perfect one and that employed by good is harmless. This is not negativity but perfect poise, a completed point of view and divine understanding."

Alice Bailey
Esoteric Healing
Fort Orange 1978

FUSION

If disease is removed, then the potential of life can occur.
However, disease, prejudice and corkscrew thinking
can also trigger the process of healing.
All are fundamental to fusion.

In the maelstrom of forces acting in the dance of life and death,
living beings need every advantage they can get.
Achieving a balance and skill-full use of experience
enables living beings to navigate successfully.
Accurate perception of the forces of fragmentation and chaos,
trauma and physical damage, allows us to choose our path.

Everything needs to be included and understood.
If any part is taken out of the equation,
distortion of the nature of our being will lead to disease.
If we can achieve balance, then healing and fusion will occur.

Wisdom may also occur.
This is a definite advantage!

"Heaven descends.
Earth ascends.
They join.
Heaven and earth mingle within the man.
The wise man brings accord to the people."

Sam Reifler
I Ching, hexagram 11, Peace
Bantam 1981

GATHERING

Plunged into awareness at birth and exposed to the twenty-first century,
filtered through where you were born,
what your family and culture and spiritual practice says,
why do certain things still attract and others repel?

Obvious answers are circumstance, ideology,
self-interest, desire, economic factors, cultural factors.
These are self-evident.
Hidden factors are also there,
ones we may refuse to acknowledge and deny to our friends
or within our cultures, and often focussed around our deepest instincts.
These are not so self-evident.

So why do people have attractions and aversions
that on the surface do not connect with obvious answers?
What really drives our motivation to live and grow?
What really happens when we suffer confusion?
What really happens when we grow and thrive?

Released from restrictions of family, culture, religion, science and morality,
where does our motivation feed?
Where will our instinct take us?

Are we really prepared to face ourselves?

"We often wonder why one child in a family differs so greatly from the
others: why, for example, among seven brothers one is so different as to
appear the antithesis of the others ... possessing traits that are not even
found in the father and mother."

Proceso Sanchez Ortega
Notes on the Miasms

GROWTH

Every living system goes through a complex cycle of growth
with each stage unfolding in a sequence.

If any part of that sequence is hindered, then disease develops.
Distortion arrests potential.
Balance is lost.
Fragmentation, collapse, even death can occur.

Life will fight for survival if motivation remains undamaged.
The potential of life and growth can overcome every obstacle,
but not in every individual case.
In health, life will naturally grow and change to reach fusion.

Anything that prevents this process is disease.

"In the healthy condition of man, the spiritual vital force, the dynamis
that animates the material body, rules with unbounded sway,
and retains all parts of the organism in admirable, harmonious, vital
operation, as regards both sensations and functions, so that our
indwelling, reason-gifted mind can freely employ this living healthy
instrument for the higher purposes of our existence."

Samuel Hahnemann
Aphorism 9, The Organon of Medicine
B Jain

HEALING

Healing has always been part of human experience.
We have survived with the planet over epochs.
It is instinctive for us.

Healing is growth.
The ability to cope with change and to leap beyond it.
We all begin as part of a group, emerging out of herd behaviour.
Most of us only use ten percent of our brain.
However, if we are lucky, we individuate and begin to grow.
Potential is always there.

Remember that pain increases as life increases.
Remember that healing can hurt more that the original trauma.
The reward is survival and fusion.
This can lead to confusion, even wisdom.

Anything that prevents this process is disease.

"The spear in the Other's heart
is the spear in your own:
you are s/he.
There is no other wisdom,
and no other hope for us
but that we grow wise."

Attributed to Surak
Star Trek
Paramount Pictures

HOPE

Kindness engenders life by its vitality and by hope.
It feels good!

Hope is kind and cruel.
Hope will reflect fragmentation and distortion as well as survival.
Seen through the mirror, hope dances like a sprite through our fate.
It does not seem to obey any laws, but it is a sign of life.

Wisdom looks fondly on hope, but it does not obey it.
However, wisdom is founded on hope and ultimately, it is governed by it.

"I am a stag, of seven tines,
I am a flood; across a plane,
I am a wind; on a deep lake,
I am a tear; the sun let fall,
I am a hawk; above the cliff,
I am a thorn; beneath the nail,
I am a wonder; among flowers,
I am a wizard; who but I sets the cool head aflame with smoke?"

The Song of Amergin
Robert Graves
The White Goddess
Faber and Faber 1975

INAPPROPRIATE TREATMENT

Regard a boil.
Is it good to let it burst?
Is it better to get the body to re-absorb the pus contained within?
(Both methods are used, where appropriate).

We often see drugs used to control
extreme emotional and mental states, even spiritual trauma.
Are they helping the boil to burst,
or helping the person to re-absorb events?
(Both methods are used where appropriate).

Things that assist us are beneficial,
unless they assist us to extremes that damage us.
Things that block us can damage us,
but they can make us adapt and change also.
Things that cut across us can be lethal,
but they can warn others to avoid the danger.
(All methods are used where appropriate).

What are we doing with antibiotics in infectious disease?
We know that a fever is the way a body fights disease,
so why do we suppress it?
How do we expect immune systems to be healthy
if they are never allowed to develop healthy reactions?
But do we leave immune systems to be overwhelmed,
knowing that we can assist with medication?
(New methods will be used where appropriate).

"Medicines should be prescribed only when they are essential, and in all cases the benefit of administering the medicine should be considered in relation to the risk involved."

General Guidelines, British National Formulary
British Medical Association and the Royal Pharmaceutical Society 1992

INSTINCT

Human behaviour has not significantly changed over the ages.
Social and cultural structures still have basic archaic roots.
Only ten percent of our brain capacity is used.
Ninety percent of our behaviour is unconscious
and most probably hundreds of thousands of years old.

What does all this mean?

Today, we court chaos.
Society and culture will have to change
under the pressure of global consciousness.

What does all this mean?

Will we keep the best from the past
or throw the human baby away with the bathwater?
Will we achieve our potential or collapse under the weight of choice?
Can we keep our motivation or will we suffer fragmentation?
Will we choose cruelty or kindness?
Will we opt for fusion and life or for death?

Note that we are still far behind our potential.
Note how much of our behaviour is unconscious.
So where does our instinct feed?

"Innate propensity, especially in lower animals to seemingly rational acts,
innate impulse, intuition. Filled, charged with life energy."

The Pocket Oxford Dictionary: 'Instinct'
1969

INTROVERT

Some of us like to withdraw and study others.
We like to be quiet and introspective.
We like to think deeply about ideas and reflect long on each issue.
We tend to take our own counsel above that of others.
This strategy bruises others who have a different approach and who
need feedback to make decisions.
They tend to become louder and more vocal around us, as their neces-
sary feedback is denied.

Each is offended by the other, even though we all use many different
strategies at different times and in different situations!

Knowing this prevents distortion and prejudice.
Knowing this prevents cruelty and corkscrew thinking.
Knowing this makes healing easier.

"Oh, if you but knew how you the purpose cherish whiles thus you mock
it! How, in stripping it, you more invest it! Ebbing men, indeed, most
often do so near to bottom run by their own fear or sloth."

William Shakespeare
The Tempest

INVASION

Invasion can occur on any level.
Physical, emotional, mental or spiritual.
It can happen in a single incident, or over years of erosion.
However, it will always affect the whole of our being.

This is the first trauma.

A second trauma results from the reaction of the person to the invasion.
A third trauma results from inappropriate reactions of others.
This includes inappropriate treatment.
When healing does not occur, this is a fourth trauma.

Obviously, other traumas may pile on top of this as well.

Too many traumas can overwhelm life.
This will trigger the process of healing, change and growth.
Or it will trigger collapse, possibly death.

"Even if cannibalism existed occasionally,
the contribution of human flesh to the diet must have been minimal and
sporadic, paling into insignificance beside that of the other creatures,
especially the big herbivores."

C Renfrew and P Bahn
Archaeology: Theories, Methods and Practice
Thames and Hudson 1996

KINDNESS

If life suffers assault or invasion, either by immediate trauma
or long-term fragmentation, the end result is disease.

Healing is an ultimate act of kindness.
Indeed, it is the key!

Functioning on all levels needs to normalise and balance.
The counterpoint reaction to disease triggers the process of healing.
Kindness prevents prejudice and corkscrew thinking and eases distortion.

Even if medical or surgical intervention is necessary,
kindness and healing are our only hope of survival.

Knowing this prevents cruelty.
Kindness sees beyond the stereotype.

"May I become at all times both now and forever
a protector for those without protection
a guide for those who have lost their way
a ship for those with oceans to cross
a bridge for those with rivers to cross
a sanctuary for those in danger
a lamp for those in need of light
a place of refuge for those in need of shelter
and a servant to all those in need."

The Dalai Lama
Ancient Wisdom, Modern World
Little, Brown and Co 1999

LANGUAGE

Human speech is extraordinarily complex.
Each language contains many different forms of speech within it.

Different language is used to describe different aspects of life.
Some forms are forbidden.
Some forms are forced to die out.
Some forms are elevated as official language.

All cultures use official language in public.
All cultures also use healing language, subjective language
and covert language.
All language forms are laced with innuendo and corkscrew
in endlessly evolving forms.

Language is alive.
We use it to determine reality.

Why else would some forms of language be forbidden?
Why else would some forms of language be elevated?

Healing language is healing ourselves.

"Now if they assert that it is idle for men's imagination to conceive of
infinite tracts of space, since there is no space beyond this World, then the
reply is: it is idle for men to imagine previous ages of God's inactivity,
since there is no time before the World began."

St Augustine
City of God
Penguin 1984

COVERT LANGUAGE

Covert language is often archaic and can contain swearing and cursing,
but it is also futuristic, being connected to growth.

Covert language is often a problem
as our internal experience rarely mirrors official realities.
It will not remain within official parameters,
seeking always to push at boundaries, to break down old structures
and to redefine human experience.
It will not tolerate the prejudice of taboo or stereotype, but it uses them.
It will use cruelty and kindness in equal measure.

Forcing life to be trapped and contained within limited language
leads to corkscrew thinking and to distortion.

We need balance here.

Healing language is healing ourselves.

"To this question the orthodox theory provides no answer – merely takes
it for granted that the defective eye is incurable and cannot, in spite of its
peculiarly intimate relationship with the psyche, be re-educated towards
normality by any process of mind-body co-ordination."

Aldous Huxley
The Art of Seeing
Chatto and Windus 1943

HEALING LANGUAGE

Language heals if it illuminates the subjective landscape of the individual,
allowing it to interface successfully with the objective world.

Often, subjective language and healing language are regarded
as covert language, because none are official language.

As life grows and changes or reacts to assault, invasion or disease,
the more difficult it is to remain within official language,
which is by nature static and unchanging.
There is a line of prejudice here that prevents healing,
as official language cannot incorporate forbidden forms.
Thus the corkscrew causes distortion of language,
which will thus contain more and more subjective,
covert and healing language.

Healing language is a response to trauma and cruelty by promoting kindness.
It promotes fusion and rejects the stereotype.
It looks underneath the sacred, the profane and the taboo.

Healing language is healing ourselves.

"... which more or less equated a civilisation with an ideology, as a zone
dominated by a prevalent 'cosmology' or model of how the World works.
This model, of course, would always be devised and imposed in the
interests of a power elite."

Felipe Fernandez Armesto
Civilisations
Macmillan 2000

OFFICIAL LANGUAGE

Official language has always been used to control ideas throughout history.

Proclaiming certain ideas or speech as heresy
is the weapon of choice for all ideologies
wishing to promote their world-view by forbidding others.

Thus official language freeze-frames evolving systems
and becomes as restrictive as an old skin.

Forcing life to become trapped and contained by limiting language
leads to corkscrew thinking and distortion of ideas.
It promotes cruelty and prejudice by pronouncing all other forms taboo.

We need balance here.
Healing language is healing ourselves.

"Words can be potent magic indeed, but they can also enslave us. We grasp from Wyrd tiny puffs of wind and store them in our lungs as words. But we may have not thereby captured a piece of reality..."

The Way of Wyrd
Brian Bates
Book Club Associates 1983

SUBJECTIVE LANGUAGE

Subjective experience is the biggest mystery
any of us will ever have to understand.

Subjective language always seems to be subject to taboo and prejudice
but mostly, it is forbidden but common parlance.
Much like swearing and cursing, 'hitting the wall',
'going down the plug hole', 'being in a hall of mirrors',
being a 'shattered mirror', 'looking into a mirror',
going through a 'plate glass window', 'withdrawing', 'going manic',
'weirding out', 'fogging out', 'being out of phase',
'being alone in a crowded room', 'being vampired',
sensing 'black shadows', 'needing psychic protection',
'pulling on an endless root', 'being in the eye of a hurricane',
'being high', 'going cosmic'.
None of this is official language.
However, language is alive and people will use it.
They will use it to define their growth and potential.
They will use it to fight cruelty, taboo and prejudice.
They will use it to create cruelty, taboo and prejudice.
We need balance here.
Healing language is healing ourselves.

"It began in what seemed in my personal narratisations as an individual
choice of a problem with which I have had an intense involvement for
most of my life: the problem of the nature and origins of all this invisible
country of touchless rememberings and unshowable reveries, this
introcosm that is more myself than anything I can find in any mirror."

Julian Jaynes
The Origins of Consciousness in the Breakdown of the Bicameral Mind
Penguin 1982

LIFE

Life is the difference between a dead body and a living one.
It is the missing link between the two.

In the dance of life and death, both states mirror each other.
Both have equal power over us.
Both states are our destiny.

Life is stronger than death.
Extinction is the agenda of death,
but note how life can be triggered by death.
Life is curious.
Its agenda is growth.
Even in death, life is thinking.

Knowing this makes healing easier.

"The material organism, without the vital force, is capable of no sensation,
no function, no self preservation; it derives all sensation and performs
all the functions of life solely by means of the immortal being (the vital
principle) which animates the material organism in health and in disease."

Samuel Hahnemann
Aphorism 10, The Organon of Medicine

MAGNETIC

Magnetic energy is soft and powerful and often disguised or subtle.
Electric energy is distorted in its presence.

However, its presence transforms us.
Its absence can remove motivation and lead to death.
Like fire, it is a good servant, but a poor master.
Under its powerful influence we can suffer great damage.
The subtlety of this energy upon living systems is grossly misunderstood.
Its effect on us is profound,
but hidden in ways that are of vital importance to our nature.
If we ignore it, we misunderstand ourselves utterly.
We pine for it, not knowing what we miss.
If we embrace it, we are in danger of distortion.

Balance is the key.

"Such traditions always contain the collective wisdom and magical
symbolism of the culture in which they developed; they often preserve
this wisdom long after its deeper aspects have been removed from formal
religion by the arrival of new cults or political restrictions."

R J Stewart
The Merlin Tarot
Aquarian 1988

MIRROR

Magnetic forces join us to our reflected image.
The reversal of reality
demonstrates the connection between the two images.
See how hard it is to separate them?

Electric charges demonstrate the presence of the connection we have
to the distortion that affects us.
See how shocking it is to separate them?

White light contains all colours, except black, which it reflects.
Black absorbs all other colours, except white, which it reflects.
Does this mean it is possible to separate them?

Does this mean that we are the Other?
Together, are we complete?

"Real contempt for the Other is a civilised vice rather than a universal
trait. The self-differentiation of the civilised is of a peculiar kind, precisely
because it is selective. People who belong to a civilisation share a sense
that their achievements set them apart from other peoples .... They are
enemies visible to each other in a kind of mirror."

Felipe Fernandez Armesto
Civilisations
Macmillan 2000

MOTIVATION

Why should we strive for life or for healing?
Why should we avoid death, if it stops pain?
Why should we change and grow if it hurts or it is hard work?

We need to know the answers or our motivation may collapse.
Building motivation can be very hard if experiences are painful and difficult.
Constant struggle damages our chance of survival,
but it can also determine our choice for life,
according to our core beliefs.
Fusion can occur if we can Balance our prejudice with healing,
our trauma with kindness and our taboo with wisdom.
We have to leap out of our stereotype!

If motivation is damaged, then healing is difficult.
This is central to survival and the choices we make.
It is important to rework equations of motivation.
We must ensure the motivation of our core being is adequate for life,
and that it will facilitate healing, change and growth.
Knowing this prevents disease.

"The first men, by all traditional accounts, lived in perfect harmony
with Nature and the gods. Of their own accord, said Ovid, without the
compulsion of Law, they were honest and true."

John Michell
The Earth Spirit
Avon 1975

PHYSICAL DAMAGE

What could damage the body?

External sources include bacteria, viruses,
foreign bodies including pollution from all sources, poisons and radiation
as well as assault, invasion and trauma from the world around us.
These are never hidden.

Internal sources include build-up of fats and toxins
and post-infective residues and effects of invasion
from the way we react to disease and the world around us.
It also includes distortion and fragmentation from corkscrew thinking,
cruelty, prejudice and taboo.
These are mostly hidden.

The exhaustion that builds up from disease and trauma
and invasion and assault over time can be catastrophic.
It can lead to collapse and physical damage.
This is always hidden.

As a completely self-repairing, self-maintaining mechanism,
a healthy body should easily last a lifetime.
Repairing and healing damage is possible if balance can be achieved.
Healing language will help.

"Many races, like many individuals, have indulged in practices
which must in the end destroy them."

J G Frazer
The Golden Bough
Macmillan 1974

POTENTIAL

You can look someone in their eye or up their arse, as you choose.
A stereotype is only the first step to understanding the Other.

Own your own dark side.
Own your own light side.
Own everything that is in between.
Avoid cruelty and distortion.
Own everything that is yours.
Blame no one, not even yourself.
Judge no one, not even yourself.

Remember to contain and safely earth
all violent consequences to safeguard life.
Remember that all actions evoke fate, which you will have to account for.
Remember that pain increases as life increases.
Remember that healing, change and growth
can hurt more than the original trauma.

Anything that prevents this understanding is disease.

"The Roman Fates and some Gaulish Mother Goddesses were perceived
to be able not only to predict the life and death of humans, but also to
terminate life by snapping the thread."

Miranda Green
Exploring the World of the Druids
Thames and Hudson 1997

PREJUDICE

Language of equality will bear reversal.
If it will not reverse, it is prejudiced.

We require a scapegoat if we need to mirror our fragmentation.
We require a scapegoat if we have suffered distortion.
We can learn so much from our Other.
The magnetic and electric connections between us
demonstrate that they are part of us.
They reflect that which we do not understand.

It is an ultimate act of cruelty to make an Other taboo.
It is a total act of invasion to use a stereotype to inflict pain.
It is an abomination to use assault and indulge in prejudice.
This is disease.

Kindness is a better law.

"Those concentration camp pictures profoundly altered my view of
so-called civilised human nature. We were certainly familiar with torture
and cruel punishments as part of history. We realised, at least theoretically,
that there was no limit to man's capacity for cruelty to man."

A Storr
Human Destructiveness
Routledge 1991

PROCESS

Most people know about boils!

First, there is pain and tenderness, swelling,
discolouration and then eruption.
No healing takes place until the discharge has occurred.
Then the boil heals from the base,
a scab forms which then drops off (more discharge).
Occasionally, the body will re-absorb the reaction
before it gets too inflamed.
The body has processed an invader.

This process is the same, whether triggered by bacterial invasion,
internal causes, psychological events or external situations.
The body makes no distinction about invasion from any source.
All are attacks on life.
Disease takes many forms, but all disease is invasion.

The process of healing will vary only in subtlety, not in form.
Even if the disease was spiritual in origin, it will still end up the toilet
once the body has finished processing it!

Knowing the process makes healing easier.

"We therefore study simple substance, in order that we may arrive at the
nature of sick-making substances. We also potentize our medicines in
order to arrive at their simple substance;
that is the nature and quality of the remedy itself."

J T Kent
Lectures on Homoeopathic Philosophy
B Jain 1986

SPIRAL

To avoid corkscrew thinking,
it is important to gather all possible information into a circle of illumination.

Every issue needs to be investigated from every angle, every dimension,
through time, through close contacts.
Every living being is in a constellation with others, we are all social beings.
From individual to culture, to society to species,
from future predictions to knowledge of origins, all must be considered.
We must try to perceive the structure of the whole.
Nothing can be left out.

Each circle of illumination is a discrete point
in the stream of consciousness.
All of these points taken together form a spiral.
Each spiral forms part of the stream of consciousness.
For true understanding, this larger picture must be grasped,
and its reflection seen as part of the dance of life and death.

Knowing this prevents disease.

"There are within every one of us three stages of knowledge.
This is the spiral process...."

Jill Purce
The Mystic Spiral
Avon 1974

STEREOTYPE

Using shorthand methods to store information is instinctive for us.
Information and communication is part of our nature.

We only use ten percent of our brain capacity,
so most of the time we use shortcuts almost exclusively.
However, reality is one hundred percent.
We do not contain it, order it or control it,
except subjectively in order to relate to it.
Thus reality is constantly tripping us up.
Unless we change and grow,
we will not meet the challenge of the future.
Shorthand methods have been of evolutionary advantage in our past,
but they will not suffice under the pressure of global consciousness.
Messing around in distortion and confusion, using corkscrew thinking
and allowing prejudice, cruelty and taboo
to form totally inadequate equations does not bode well for our species.
We need to evolve or die!

"A fire burns at the foot of the mountain.
The superior man is brilliant as an administrator,
but he dare not act as a judge."

Sam Reifler
I Ching, hexagram 22, Beauty
Bantam 1981

SURVIVAL

Life is preset to achieve its potential, deep in the genus species.
Motivation is constantly updated and can easily be damaged.
Disease will interfere with this process.

If distortion, fragmentation and disease constantly prevent balance,
life may construct a different equation.
Healing may not be judged worth the pain or the effort.
Easing pain through death may seem a better option.
Sometimes death is chosen instead of life.
This is a result of disease and trauma.

However, by occurring, disease can trigger
the magnetic reversal of death energy.
Thus through the mirror, life energy is fortified.
Fusion is possible if kindness is understood.

Knowing the process makes healing easier.

"The pain is too much.
A thousand grim winters grow in my head.
In my ears the sound of the coming dead.
All seasons.
All sane.
All living.
All pain.
No opiate to lock still my senses,
Only left the body locked tenses."

Spike Milligan and A Clare
Depression and How to Survive It
Arrowhead 1994

TABOO

History and archaeology show us that we are naturally violent.
Powerful ideas have never baulked at eradicating opposition.
Some things are allowed, others aren't.
This line defines the sacred, the profane and the taboo.

People like to be individual and part of a herd, all at the same time.
We like to extend our boundaries and to remain within our identity.
We all like to exclude the Other in order to define ourselves.
The corkscrew inflames prejudice and concepts of the Other.
This causes trauma.
Scapegoats and stereotypes reflect our cruelty.
They mirror our distortion.
Confusion indulges in fragmentation.
This will result in disease.
This is the result of disease.
Is it the fate of our species to prefer death or life?

"Moreover, witnesses – if there are any – can be heard against such an individual. He himself can be constrained in various ways including limitation of food and being held in chains. He can even, on the recommendation of qualified persons, to be put to the question is order to get at the truth, as the nature of the business at hand and the condition of the person may require."

Bernard Gui
The Inquisitors Manual
H C Lea, A History of the Inquisition of the Middle Ages
Harper and Bros 1887

TRAUMA

Any invasion or assault on life results in fragmentation and distortion.
The effect is a counter-reaction of confusion and healing.
Each is a mirror of the other.
This will cause change and growth, or collapse, even death.

Any invasion or assault on life will affect all levels, physical, emotional,
mental or spiritual, no matter which of these levels it directly impacts.
It is a shockwave rippling out, causing disease.
It is not always possible to judge which eventuality will win out.
But life is stronger than death, as long as motivation is in balance.

Wisdom and kindness indicate healing, detoxification
and common sense procedures are the only way out of this pain.
Inappropriate treatment can still result in trauma.
Exhaustion and physical damage can still lead to collapse, even death.

"... the central disturbance, as we called it, comes first
and this is followed by changes in various organ systems depending on
each individual's pathological tendencies. Pathology grows on the central
disturbance like a creeper on a stick. What we have to do is remove the
central disturbance."

Rajan Sankaran
The Substance of Homoeopathy
Homoeopathic Medical Publishers 1994

WHITE

White incorporates all colours, but as it absorbs them, it obscures them.
White has a vibration that energises life.
It reduces complexity and enables simplicity.
It is clean and pure and restful.
Thus hope springs from this focus of clarity.
This focus is experienced as oneness.
It releases energy and enthusiasm.
It invigorates motivation.
This purity generates electric and magnetic energy.
It is a mirror to survival.
This focus is a balance to chaos.
It is thus restful and allows fusion.
However, it cannot sustain growth.
This bright point of focus obscures difference.
It obscures colours and so cannot sustain life,
which depends upon diversity to flourish.
White energy is thus used to form a focal point around momentary clarity,
allowing instinct to leap into wisdom through confusion.

"I looked then and saw that his robes, which had seemed white, were not
so, but were woven of all colours, and if he moved they shimmered and
changed hue so that the eye was bewildered.
'I liked white better,' I said.
'White!' he sneered. 'It serves as a beginning. White cloth may be dyed.
The white page can be overwritten; and the white light can be broken.'
'In which case it is no longer white,' said I. 'And he that breaks a thing to
find out what it is has left the path of wisdom.'

J R R Tolkien
The Fellowship of the Ring: The Council of Elrond
George Allen and Unwin 1969

WISDOM

Black, white and red are primal ancestral colours
from the very roots of our beginning.
The number *three* is also present in our origin.
White, red and black combine in infinite and intricate subtlety
in the dance of life and death.
Wisdom requires that all factors be considered.
Nothing can be lost!
All must be included in the whole.
All of the grey areas, plus both sides of all of the arguments, in all of the
continuums of all the ideas that exist, have existed or can become possible.
Also, all of those things that don't exist,
have never existed and may not be possible must be considered.
We need to come to grips with our nature
and learn to set our motivation to achieve our potential.
There is no possibility of balance if anything is left out of our equations.
Though we may deny and negate or disavow, things exist despite our actions.
We have simply distorted our perception for subjective reasons
or emotional contentment or mental peace or spiritual satisfaction.
Do we really want to live within our own reality, never to be allowed out?
Don't we all want choices?
Would we accept any one else determining our reality?
Don't we all want to be included?
What happens to that which we exclude?
What happens to that which we include?

"It has become abundantly clear that human behaviour is active in
character, but that it is determined not only be past experience, but also
by plans and designs formulating the future, and that the human brain is a
remarkable apparatus which cannot only create these models of the future,
but also subordinates its behaviour to them."

A R Luria
The Working Brain: An Introduction to Neuropsychology
Penguin 1981

"The physician's high and only mission is to restore the sick to health, to cure, as it is termed.
The highest idea of cure is rapid, gentle and permanent restoration of the health, or removal and annihilation of the disease in its whole extent, in the shortest, most reliable, and most harmless way, on easily comprehensible principles.
If the physician clearly perceives what is to be cured in disease ... if he clearly perceives what is curative in medicines ... "

Samuel Hahnemann
Aphorisms 1, 2, 3, The Organon of Medicine

THE LOST RED BOOK OF HEALING

To my father.

Strength.
"You have always been strong.
You were the strongest force in my universe.
You embody life's potential.
The past lives within you.
It has formed you.
You built our future."

January 2002

In order to achieve strength, we need to take our awareness,
grow to our full potential, and then extend out into the universe.

Anything that prevents this process is an enemy or a friend.

AWARENESS

For aeons we have sought awareness.
We study and sacrifice, scrimp and save,
spend and bankrupt ourselves in its pursuit.

But a small child has awareness; so do the lilies of the field.
All life has awareness.
If we can understand this, we can relax and enter its state.
This will allow strength to grow, distortion to fade,
and it will stabilise our language of power.
It will allow us to see what potential we have.
It will allow us to evolve
and resist the imprint of past trauma turning us to hate.
It can do all of this if we balance awareness
with knowledge and the wisdom to understand.
This is the most important manoeuvre in the process of healing.
This is the most important escape we will ever achieve.
This is the most important component of freedom.

Its simplicity has always kept it hidden.

"For winter's rain and ruins are over,
and all the season of snow and sins;
The days divided lover and lover,
The light that loses, the night that wins,
And time remembered in grief forgotten,
And frosts are slain and flowers begotten,
And in green underwood and cover
Blossom by blossom the spring begins."

Atalanta in Caydon
Algernon Swinburne
William Heinemann 1923

BALANCE

From the maelstrom we emerge into a spinning universe.
Chaos and justice compete
as life and death spiral into change and growth.

What do we want, what do we need, what will enable us?
What will we do with the healing and the freedom we have won
through our potential and our strength?

Laws determine structure.
The only constant is change.
We can only achieve balance momentarily, before the circle moves us on.
Stasis is death, so we must plunge back into the maelstrom, as fate dictates.

However, once we have attained balance,
though we lose it again, we can recognise it.
This is balance!
This is wisdom!

Anything that prevents this process is an enemy.

"We unleash at long last the full, unbridled power of human diversity on
our planet's prolific problems. The outcome of this gender awakening will
be a new species, a new humanity; one that has as its fundamental purpose
the assurance of a healthy and fulfilling life time as a birthright for all."

Martine Rothblatt
The Apartheid of Sex
HarperCollins 1996

CHANGE

The only constant in the universe is change.
Nothing stays the same.

With balance, fusion and healing, we can become strong.
We learn to avoid trauma, as we understand the imprint of the past.
Growth demands change.
We cannot stay in stasis where disease is the rule.
We know how to move and change direction now.
If we can give ourselves permission to enter the process of healing,
we can complete a manoeuvre.
If we can do it once, we can do it again.
We can explore our environment by doing it again.
This is language of power!

The circle turns, the spiral spins,
the stream of consciousness moves imperceptibly.

Fate now has the strength to evolve, as we escape from trauma.

"While recovery from an individual symptom often takes place, the
constitution which is the basis of the hysterical reaction to difficulties
remains in most cases. Sometimes a hysterical symptom lasts indefinitely
because the situation to which it is a reaction also persists e.g. in a patient
who has developed hysterical symptoms after an injury which entitles him
to compensation."

Sir Roger Bannister
Brain's Clinical Neurology
Oxford University Press 1985

CHAOS

Chaos has to be experienced!
We can go into it and come out of it
according to the permission we give our motivation and our direction,
according to which manoeuvre we wish to carry out.

Once we understand the process of healing and disease,
we can change our language of weakness and learn the language of power.
Then we can reach for strength.

Once we taste strength, we can reach for freedom.
Once we reach for freedom, we can feel joy.
Spinning through the universe, we can escape from distortion.

As soon as we find balance, change dictates that we enter chaos again!

If you find yourself falling, you may as well learn how to fly!

"The only flaw is that in order for me to have a different orderly view of
the world and myself, a view even more suited to my temperament, I have
to walk along the edge of the abyss, and I have doubts that I have the
daring and strength to accomplish that feat. But who is there to tell?"

Carlos Casteneda
The Wheel of Time
Penguin 1987

CIRCLE

To avoid distortion and trauma, it is important
to gather all possible information into a circle of illumination.

Language of weakness leads to weak ideas and weak thoughts.
Strength dictates that our minds grow resolute in the service of the future.
Language of power is required to obtain permission
to complete the manoeuvre of the process of healing.
This turns the circle of life and death
and spins the magnetic and electric energy that creates the universe.

Joy is the child of freedom.
Justice is the child of wisdom.

We can choose our direction and motivation to avoid chaos.
We have the potential to understand our fate.
Do we have the balance to ensure survival?

"No wonder that it was so well guarded in the inner mysteries as the
source of the different teachings given out from time to time, veiled
in numerous ways and under symbols and allegories, in case it might
be misunderstood by those not yet sufficiently developed mentally and
morally, and therefore ready to condemn and destroy."

W P Rigg
Astrology of the Mysteries
Private publication

COLLAPSE

Sometimes life lives!
Sometimes it will resist distortion.
Sometimes it will save all its parts and find balance.

Each collapse is a mirror to the possibilities it contains.
The reflection forms part of the dance of life and death.
Its forms are infinite.

Survival is sometimes the outcome.
Equations will be finely worked.
The circle turns, the spiral spins and fate intervenes.
The stream of consciousness continues.
Electric and magnetic charges flicker around the scene.

Strength forms as freedom is experienced.
Joy flows into wisdom.

"Just how brave the author is to challenge the establishment might not be appreciated by those of us who do not live in America. He has challenged the powerful and prestigious profession of psychiatry, the immensely wealthy and influential drug industry, and that vast number of people who prefer to believe that there are such things as mental illnesses rather than to take responsibility for their own lives and for the influence that they have on their children. This is heresy."

Peter Breggin
Toxic Psychiatry
HarperCollins 1993

COMMON SENSE PROCEDURES

Find at least three people you can confide and communicate with
for support during the healing and recovery process.
Don't be afraid to extend this basic structure
to others who are prepared to help.
This is called a three-legged stool.
It will allow you to gain strength by learning the language of power.
It will help you to understand the language of weakness
and where this will ultimately lead you.
Do this quickly!

Practice balance and joy.
Study what kind of manoeuvre and permission you need
to gain awareness and wisdom.
Do everything you can to help your body to find healing.
Do this for the rest of your life!

"Excessive vivacity follows the use of strong coffee (primary reaction), but
sluggishness and drowsiness remain for a long time afterwards
(secondary reaction), if this be not always again removed for a short
time by imbibing fresh supplies of coffee (palliative). After the profound
stupefied sleep caused by opium (primary reaction), the following
night will be all the more sleepless (secondary reaction). After all the
constipation produced by opium (primary reaction), diarrhoea ensues
(secondary reaction); and after purgation with medicines that irritate the
bowels, constipation of several days duration ensues (secondary reaction)."

Samuel Hahnemann
Aphorism 65, The Organon of Medicine

DEATH

Death is part of life.
We are infinite creatures!

Death of an old idea, a way of being, a mode of thinking, a basis of belief,
will lead to new beginnings.
Thus we can attempt change and growth and potential.
We must understand our true nature, or our equations will be inadequate.
Our strategies will always be weak
if we do not understand the baby in our bathwater.
Our language will never be strong or incisive or of any use to us at all!
Language of weakness will always work against us
and we will be our own enemy.
Thus, we will cause our own trauma and damage our own survival.
Freedom dictates that we have this choice.
Our actions will trigger fate.
Freedom dictates that we have other choices too.
These will also trigger fate.
Direction is crucial.

Understanding this manoeuvre depends on our motivation.

Joy is the key!

"Pasteur made a wise remark when he called upon the verdict of time
to pass sentence on a scientist. As a matter of fact, Bechamp, with the
assurance of genius, never lost hope in this final judgement."

Ethel Douglas Hume
Pasteur Exposed
Bookreal 1989

DIRECTION

Achieving balance and fusion is one thing!
What next?
In order to complete a manoeuvre, we have to decide on a direction.
Poised at the point of balance and fusion, we have to change.
Poised at the point of permission and understanding, we have to evolve!
Do we go back into chaos?
Do we go back into the past?
Do we go forward into the future?
Do we go forward into wisdom?
Do we accept the now?
Do we give ourselves permission to circle and spiral.
Do we try for joy?
Or do we collapse into disease, back into the spinning universe?
What does your motivation say?
Life or death?
Strength or disease?
Enemy or friend?
Love or hate?

"During the past year another major fact has become apparent. The key names have broken down into two groups on a geographical basis. The names in the first group, which appear to be older, are all to be found in all parts of the world ... the most logical conclusion is that in prehistoric times instead of one there were two dispersals from the Mediterranean ..."

John Cohane
The Key
Fontana 1975

DISEASE

Disease changes life.
It causes spinning and trauma.
It causes alteration and fluctuation in life.
In the body, the process is seen via symptoms.
In the emotions, chaos can be observed.
In the mind, intellectual processes struggle.
In the spirit, distortion is evident.
Disease is observable as a shockwave rippling out.
Then a secondary reaction from life occurs.
Life spins on all levels.
This distortion can be obvious or subtle.
Disease takes many forms.
The reaction of life in response is equally complex.
Many complex continuums interact.
Kindness is the key!
Understand this!
This is strength!

"In part the themes and the evidence in this book do suggest a number of conspiracies. These have been acted out in secret by groups of people on behalf of vested interests. More profoundly, though, the evidence suggests a cultural concordance, an invisible mix of minute and everyday contracts of cultural, political and economic orthodoxy.
To be a party to such a hegemony, people do not have to conspire, they need not even be in contact with each other."

Martin Walker
Dirty Medicine
Slingshot 1994

DISTORTION

Distorted functioning on any level can quickly lead to disease.
Subtle change will eventually be as devastating as major change.
Distortion of out-moded states can be good news in some cases.
In others, it is worrying!
Vital changes can be as subtle as major changes.
This is a dangerous time!
We have to change and grow if we are to evolve.
We have to find strength and joy.
By going through the process of healing, we learn to manoeuvre.
Now, we can set our direction.
Now, we can set our motivation.
Now, we can circle and spiral around our environment.
Things still seem distorted.
Who is our friend?
Who is our enemy?
Things still seem chaotic.
Who do we love?
Who do we hate?
What do you give yourself permission to do?
Freedom dictates that we can do anything now.

"It appears that he was sitting in his quarters one evening with his
two dogs. They suddenly became disturbed and began to investigate
something that wasn't there. He heard a voice saying distinctly to his inner
ear that I should come and ask his help and that he was to give it. He was
so impressed by this occurrence that he went to a mutual friend and asked
her whether I was in trouble of any sort. At his request she wrote to me to
enquire how I was faring, but mentioned no names, and I, not realising the
significance of the incident, returned a non-committal answer."

Don Fortune
Psychic Self Defence
Aquarian 1986

ELECTRIC

Electric energy is powerful.
It is either there or it is not there.
Magnetic energy dances in the aftermath.

It can easily cause distortion.
Its absence will reduce motivation and can cause collapse.
Its presence causes potential, the possibility of escape.
The potential of electric energy in living beings is possible to understand.
Its effect on us is strength, but hidden in ways that are vital to our nature.
Is it our servant or our master?
Understanding the gain, we could balance ourselves in its presence.
We must not embrace it, but we must learn from it and find joy.
Spinning is the key.

"Pains are very numerous; biting, boring, bruised, burning external and internal, cutting, pressing external and internal, stitching, tearing in muscles and nerves. Paralysis one-sided of organs, painless. External and internal pulsation. Pulse; fast, intermittent, irregular, small, weak. He desires to be rubbed and most symptoms are ameliorated by rubbing. Sensitiveness prevails throughout the whole proving especially to pain. Electric shocks are quite common."

J T Kent
Zincum Phosphoricum, Lectures on Homoeopathic Materia Medica
Homoeopathic Publications 1988

ENEMY

The enemy is different from the Other.
The Other is just different from us,
and only becomes an enemy when we feel threatened.
This threat may be real or imagined,
but it will trigger an automatic reaction from us.
Initially, it will cause trauma, then it will cause growth and change.
Or it will trigger disease, collapse and death.

Thus is can be understood that we have to be careful around an enemy.
It can also be understood that an enemy can ensure our survival
by changing us and facilitating our growth.

Knowing when to make an enemy of a friend or a friend of an enemy
is a mark of strength.
We need to understand that this can lead to wisdom,
and it is part of the process of healing.

"The chance for the Bishops of Rome came when Emperor Constantine
adopted the Christian faith in the fourth century, and gave them political
and legal authority, which they used to enforce their position. The ultimate
defeat of Alexandria then followed at the time of Emperor Theodosius I,
when Theophilus, his Bishop in Alexandria, destroyed the Serapeum and the
religious centre of the empire hence forward moved to the Vatican in Rome."

Ahmed Osman
Out of Egypt
Arrow 1999

ENVIRONMENT

What we believe sets our environment.
What we think dictates what we get.

We speak the language of weakness.
We believe we have no power, and so our lands are polluted.
We believe we have no permission, and so our waters stink.
We believe we cannot set our direction, and so our air poisons us.

If we learn the language of power, will our lands become clean?
If we give ourselves permission, will our waters be fit to drink?
If we take over our own direction, will our air nourish us?

But where are we all going?
What do we all want?

"The Goddess is now returning. Denied and suppressed for thousands of years of masculine domination, she comes at a time of dire need. For we walk through the valley of shadow of nuclear annihilation, and we do fear evil."

Edward Whitmont
The Return of the Goddess
Arkana 1987

ESCAPE

Remember that escape is no guarantee of survival.
Remember that healing can hurt more than the original trauma.
Indeed it is the mirror image of it.
Coming back through the mirror
only enables you to deal with the current situation.

Balance is the key!

In order to complete this manoeuvre, we have meet our fate.
In order to achieve healing and reach our potential,
we have to meet the universe.

Anything that prevents this process is an enemy.

"So she went to the brook which flowed through the garden, and drew up a pail of water full of little fish; and, at night, when the young prince was asleep, his bride drew away the covering and poured the pail of cold water and little fishes over him, so that they slipped all about him. Then the prince woke up directly, calling out; 'Oh! That makes me shiver! Dear wife, that makes me shiver! Yes, now I know what shivering means.' "

A Tale of One who Travelled to Learn what Shivering Means
Fairy Tales of Grimm
Wells Gardner Darton and Co 1948

EVOLVE

We started out as primitive creatures with a spark,
an environmental advantage.
Using this advantage we have evolved and become dominant.
We are not the only species that have done this,
and we won't be the last.

Nature changes.
It is an illusion to think that we control the forces of the universe.
Nature changes.
It is distortion that allows us to think that we dictate reality.
No matter what forces we learn to play with,
we are not in a form that can play on equal terms.
No matter how clever we think we are,
we are far from our potential, far from wisdom.

Mostly, we are egos on legs.
Pompous little creatures who think we can invent gods to protect us.
When our gods fail, we invent bombs.
When our bombs fail, what will we invent then?

"Looking back at the past four million years should make us humble
in the face of the next four million. There is every possibility that our
species will still be here at the end of that time, but whose great-great
grandchildren will be represented is anybody's guess. In the West,
personal biological reproduction is no longer a cultural imperative."

Timothy Taylor
The Prehistory of Sex
Clays 1977

FATE

Okay, so who claims to understand fate?
Mostly, we are always told in dark terms that no one can!
Ever!
This is language of weakness.
It does not enable us.
It does not inform us.
It keeps us in our place.
It stops us trying.
It does not imply permission.
If we use language of power, we can try to understand.
We can use what we know, what we think we know.
We can use things that may help, that may be relevant, that may be
completely useless, but we can put them on our palate nonetheless!
If we never try to understand our fate, we will never do so.
If we try to understand our fate, we may get it wrong,
but eventually, we will gain some awareness of it.
Once we begin to do this, we may begin to see through the glass darkly.
We will have reached the mirror.
It is a start!

"This journey back to our cultural origins has unearthed some surprising results. That cultural activities such as the making of oriental rugs, the use of the dreaded dentist's drill and the equally dreaded practice of accountancy have all been shown to be part of Neolithic life is remarkable enough ... each of the elements of civilisation has been shown to have been highly developed long before the rise of ancient Egypt and Mesopotamia."

Richard Rudgley
Lost Civilisations of the Stone Age
Arrow 1999

FREEDOM

Most people are frightened of freedom.
We are social creatures.
Most of us mythologise about freedom because we do not have it.
We are constrained by our social conditions.
Most societies fight about freedom, but none provide it totally.
If I am free, who does my work?
If I do my work, are others free?
If I take a slave, who is the slave?
If I am free, are others also free?
Free to do what?
To think my own thoughts?
If we all become free, where is culture?
Where is society?
Can I assume my culture is your culture?
Can I assume my society is your society?
Could we cope with billions of different models?
Would we overlap?
What if we all want different things?
What if we all want the same things?
This is the assumption isn't it?
Justice is the key.

"The observed diversity was, of course, due not only to the splitting of a few immigrant societies and foreign traditions. Divergence was accelerated and emphasised also on the one hand by the multiplicity of pre-existing Mesolithic groups who absorbed the Neolithic techniques or were absorbed in the Neolithic societies, on the other by the plurality of external stimuli that impinged upon them from Africa, the Levant, Anatolia and perhaps Central Asia."

V Gordon Childe
The Dawn of European Civilisation
Paladin 1973

FRIEND

A friend is different from the Other.
The Other is just different from us,
and only becomes a friend when we feel flattered.

This flattery can be real or imagined,
but it will trigger an automatic reaction from us.
Initially, it will cause joy.
Then it will trigger magnetic energy, distortion and change.
Or, will it trigger chaos, collapse and the language of weakness?

Thus it can be seen that we have to be careful around a friend.
It can also be understood that a friend can ensure our survival
by challenging us and facilitating growth.

Knowing when to make a friend of an enemy or an enemy of a friend
is a mark of strength.
We need to understand this can lead to wisdom,
and it is part of the process of healing.

"... I made a deal with her; I would repeat all the stories and myths and
legends told by man, and at the same time Lilith would have her way.
She anointed her body with oil and danced naked in the desert before an
open fire. She danced, I watched, until I felt the meaning of her
movements in my own body and soul. Only then could I begin to write
of Lilith and the children of Eve."

Barbara Black Koltov
The Book of Lilith
Nicholas Hays 1986

FUTURE

In order to have a future,
we need to ensure that we have the means to guarantee life.

It is not just a matter of knowing how to manoeuvre.
It is not enough that we have knowledge of our survival
through countless epochs.
If future conditions are completely different from anything that has gone
before, we will need to change and grow, and even evolve.

We can only evolve if we achieve the strength
to keep the past in balance with the future.
If we do anything else, we lose our identity as a genus species.
If we lose our identity, we enter chaos,
which will cause trauma and disease.

What of our future then?

"We can get outside the universe. I mean in the sense of putting a model
of the universe inside our skulls. Not a superstitious, small-minded,
parochial model filled with spirits and hobgoblins, astrology and magic,
glittering with fake crocks of gold where the rainbow ends."

Richard Dawkins
Unweaving the Rainbow
Penguin 1998

GROWTH

Every living system goes through a complex cycle of growth.
Each stage unfolds in a sequence.

We learn to avoid trauma and learn to use the language of power.
We understand we need a full palate to create our equations.
We begin manoeuvre as we become aware of joy and freedom.

This is strength!
Life will fight for survival.
Motivation learns the process of healing.
It will discover direction.
Life will successfully complete the manoeuvre of escape.
Life will take permission to explore the environment.
Life will find freedom.
Thus growth is stimulated and causes change and distortion.
Chaos is never far away,
but we can judge our progress in the mirror of wisdom.

This is wisdom!

" 'There are many things I would not do,' said Palinor. 'But no misdeed
could be graver, it seems to me, than trying to increase one's own
luminance by quenching the light shining from another ...' "

Knowledge of Angels
Jill Paton Walsh
QPD/Colt 1994

HATE

Hate is blind.
It does not see into the circle of illumination.
The grand scheme of the universe suffers distortion,
allowing an enemy to arise.

Thus, language of power is spinning into chaos.
Language of weakness reverses justice.
The spiral collapses.
Friend and enemy stare at each other through the mirror,
killing joy and revelling in trauma.

No permission to use common sense procedures is allowed.
Healing and growth are freeze-framed into disease.
Escape is not desired, but it is fought for.
Freedom, though desirable is not sought.
The past assumes a superior position.
The imprint of pain festers and poisons the environment.

We have sold our ability to understand
in order to satisfy our passion for love.

"We can thus conceive of the nature of mind in terms of the water in a lake.
When the water is stirred up by a storm, the mud from the lake's bottom
clouds it, making it appear opaque. But the nature of water is not dirty.
When the storm passes, the mind settles and the water is left clear once again."

The Dalai Lama
Ancient Wisdom, Modern World
Little, Brown and Co 1999

HEALING

Healing has always been part of human experience.
We have survived with the planet over epochs.
It is instinctive for us.

The process of healing is a manoeuvre automatically triggered by distortion.
This always triggers change, and through the mirror,
the reaction of life in response can be seen.

Thus we learn to dance with the universe,
gaining strength and confidence.
We know how to use our palate of understanding.
We know we have to search for justice.
We know we have to discover wisdom.
We know how to use balance as a fulcrum to change our direction.
We understand we must allow ourselves permission
to use language of power to approach our potential.

This is a really deep awareness of what healing can ultimately do.

"Gaulish gods in the Roman period were sometimes shown with three
faces; although others of an earlier date are only represented with two.
The Mother Goddesses, Matronae, are normally shown in groups of three.
In other words, whatever the god or goddess happened to be called, he or
she was at one time part of a trinity representing youth, middle age and
age, corresponding to the three phases of the moon."

T C Lethbridge
Gogmagog
Book Club Associates 1975

IMPRINT

Not all assaults are bad.
Not all distortion is disease.

Strength and growth need a stimulus or they will not occur.
Love may cause change, but so will hate.
We may require both!
What doesn't kill us makes us stronger.

However, the imprint of previous assaults and the resultant distortions
of disease will eventually resolve like bruising coming out,
allowing the original trauma to resolve.
This process often shows time delays, as stuck impacts release,
often years later in the presence of similar experiences in the environment.
Good or bad, these old traumas are eventually given up
as we come back through the mirror.
Like the soil, we give up our secrets
as we complete the manoeuvre of healing and escape our past.
All that we require is the permission to understand our potential.

"To form a nucleus of the universal brotherhood of humanity,
without distinction of race, creed, sex, caste or colour.
To encourage the study of comparative religion, philosophy and science.
To investigate unexplained laws of nature and the powers latent in man."

H P Blavatsky
The Theosophical Society 1875
The Secret Doctrine
First Quest 1967

INAPPROPRIATE TREATMENT

Things that assist us are beneficial,
unless they assist us to extremes that damage us.
Balance is the key.

Matching individual circumstances with appropriate treatment
gives us a better chance to enable to process of healing.

Remember that all methods are appropriate in individual circumstances.
Remember that all methods can imprint the process.
Permission to use the language of power can spin trauma into freedom.

Thus as we unlearn the pattern of disease.
Joy will ease trauma.
Justice will ease chaos.
Awareness can lead to wisdom.

"The drugs synthesised since the end of World War II have achieved their
end – the antibiotic sterilisation, more or less, of patient's bodies – at the
expense of the immune system, and AIDS is the last stop in the line. The
immune system cannot be suppressed and undermined indefinitely
without a price being paid. The chickens have come home to roost."

Harris Coulter
Aids and Syphilis: The Hidden Link
North Atlantic 1987

JOY

If we satisfy our appetites, this gives us joy.
However, appetites can become satiated; they often do.
Then they change as we become bored with them.

If we find love, this gives us joy.
However, love can become fulfilled, it often does.
Then it can change and we feel differently.

If we find hate, this gives us joy.
However, hate can become jaded; it often does.
Then it can change and we tire of it.

If we find wisdom, will this give us joy?
As no one ever really has, who can tell?
Wisdom is an appetite that can never be really satiated.
It cannot become jaded.
It cannot be satisfied.
Is this why it gives us joy!

"Will the unicorn be willing to serve thee, or abide by thy crib? Canst
thou bind the unicorn with his band in the furrow? Or will he harrow the
valleys after thee? Wilt thou leave thy labour to him ...?"

Kathleen Raine
Blake and Antiquity
Routledge and Keegan Paul 1979

JUSTICE

If we conquer our appetites, is this justice?
Do we really only need justice to keep the urge for life contained?

If we allow freedom, will this equal justice?
All those multitudinous differences all allowed?
All those billions of individual freedoms,
competing for resources in the environment?

If we allow wisdom, will this enable justice?
All those multitudinous individuals spinning in the universe
competing for resources.
All those appetites needing to be satisfied?
All seeking joy?

Justice is all we have until we find wisdom!
All else is chaos!

"Few books have given rise to so much misconception as the City of God.
By some it is thought to give a philosophy, by others a theology of history.
By some it is thought to contain well developed political theories, to be
hostile to the state as such and in particular to the Roman Empire, and
to outline the provinces of an established church and Christian state. By
others it is considered to be primarily a Christian reply to the charge that
Rome has been sacked because it had become Christian, as identifying the
City of God with the church, and as teaching that justice does not enter
into the definition of state."

St Augustine
City of God
Penguin 1984

LANGUAGE OF POWER

Know that language is alive, that it is a tool, and can be used as a tool!

Language of power is very old, but its aims are in the future.
It can illuminate the subjective landscape of living beings,
allowing the strength of potential to manifest.

Different forms of language allow different possibilities of survival.
It can alter the environment, allowing life to thrive.
It can allow justice, permission, awareness and freedom.
It can enable us to grasp the universe as we evolve and change.
It can remove or deny such permission, allowing disease to take hold.

The more we include on our palate, the more we allow growth.
The less we include, the more we suffer distortion.

Beware of the dark side of the force!

"For, apart from the fact that the thick fog of folly and ignorance has so
blinded our mind that it is incapable of feeling or saying anything divinely
inspired, the realisation of all our sins above all else prevails upon us to
believe that this fog might conceal even any light that our minds could
possibly possess; thus it comes about that, besides not having anything
to say, we cannot offer with any confidence even what we have, if our
conscience prevents us."

B R Rees
Pelagius On the Christian Life
Boydell 1998

LANGUAGE OF WEAKNESS

Know that language is alive, that it is a tool, and can be used as a tool!

Language of weakness is relatively modern, and its aims are all about fear.

In the distant past, people used language of power
to create a subjective impression of equality with natural forces.
They did this naturally.
In historical times, people have been forced into language of weakness,
allowing others to grasp power through distortion, hate,
trauma and assault, disease, chaos and death.

Thus language of weakness has been taught to us by an enemy!
We must grasp our own permission to develop language of power.
Thus we realise that our enemy is really our friend,
because we might not have done it without them!

"True poetic practice implies a mind so miraculously attuned and
illuminated that it can form words, by a chain of more-than-coincidences,
into a living entity – a poem that goes about on its own (for centuries after
the author's death, perhaps) affecting readers with its stored magic."

Robert Graves
The White Goddess
Faber and Faber 1975

LIFE

In the dance of life and death, both states mirror each other.
Both have equal power over us.
Both states are our destiny.

Life is stronger than death; even in death, life is thinking.

When life is given permission, it will change and grow.
Searching for joy, we sense freedom.
Searching for freedom, we find justice.
Searching for justice, we become aware of wisdom.
Searching for wisdom, we find understanding.
Searching for understanding, we escape from trauma.

Balance pivots trauma and wisdom.
As we glimpse it, we plunge back into chaos.
We can sense the spinning.
Armed with our palate, we enter the process again.
Facing the future, we face our fate and evolve.

"Movements and migrations of peoples are no longer acceptable as
explanations for the changes seen in the archaeological records. And the
very notion of discrete archaeological cultures as representing recognisable,
socially related groups of people is increasingly coming into question."

Colin Renfrew
Before Civilisation
Pimlico 1999

LOVE

Love is a blind state.
It does not see into the spiral of consciousness.
The grand scheme of the future suffers distortion,
allowing a friend to appear.

Chaos overwhelms balance, spinning into permission.
This reverses justice, but it causes a circle of growth.
Enemy and friend stare at each other through the mirror,
revelling in joy and removing freedom.
Permission is allowed, but common sense procedures
are freeze-framed into justice.
Escape is suddenly not desired.
Freedom, though desirable, is not sought.
The future assumes a superior position,
leaving the imprint of pain unaddressed.
This will undermine the environment by distorting growth and balance.
Language subtly alters, reducing permission.
We have sold our ability to achieve strength
in order to satisfy our passion for hate.

"A deep sadness also informed Augustine's later work: the fall of Rome influenced his doctrine of original sin, which would become central to the way Western people would view the world. Augustine believed that God had condemned humanity to an eternal damnation, simply because of Adam's one sin. The inherited guilt was passed on to all his descendants through the sexual act, which was polluted by what Augustine called 'concupiscence'. Concupiscence was the irrational desire to take pleasure in mere creatures instead of God."

Karen Armstrong
A History of God
Mandarin 1993

MAGNETIC

Magnetic energy can appear as a friend.
It is often distorted in our presence, just as it distorts us.
Electric energy is sent spinning and flashing all about.

Its very nature causes us to change.
Its absence causes trauma and collapse.
Is it our servant or our master, underlying both strength and joy?

The imprint of this energy on living beings is possible to understand.
Its effect on us is electric,
and obvious in ways that are vital to our nature.
We must manoeuvre ourselves, knowing what is possible.
We must not embrace it.
We must learn from it and find wisdom.

The spiral is the key.

"In concluding this part of our subject we may observe ... that fire festivals
are sun charms or magic ceremonies intended to secure a proper supply
of sunshine for men, animals and plants. He further considered that the
custom of carrying lighted brands around the fields for the purpose of
ensuring their fertility clearly shows these fires to have been mock suns."

T F G Dexter
Fire Worship in Britain
Watts and Co 1931

MANOEUVRE

In health, life has balance and motivation.
It is achieving its potential.

Direction is now vital.

If life is not healthy,
then disease and trauma will trigger the process of change and growth.
If growth has no freedom, then trauma will trigger change.
If change has no permission, then survival is threatened.

Thus it can be seen that growth, freedom and permission
are vital elements of any manoeuvre we attempt
to seek our way out of the imprint of disease.

"Although in later times the maze seems to have degenerated into a
child's game ... or provided some fun on high-days and holidays, originally
it must have been of profound significance in the initiatory ceremonies of
the Neolithic culture and may have been instrumental in raising the subtle
life-giving energies inherent in the body of the earth by means of a formal
dance paced out along the intricacies of the winding path."

Janet and Colin Bord
Mysterious Britain
Paladin 1976

MIRROR

Electric energy is discharged as we enter and leave states of distortion.
Fear of this energy glues us into our disease states.
Magnetic energy keeps us stuck in our distortion, within our appetites,
within our needs, our wants, our desires.
Fear of this attraction to trauma forces us into a tunnel
of fewer and fewer choices.
It triggers the need to escape, the hunger for freedom.
This desperate need to break free results in understanding and awareness.

If change is strangled, the balance between the opposing forces
in the mirror cause electric energy to suddenly discharge.
This is the only thing that will alter the magnetic glue
enough to allow us to escape.

Shocking as this is, it illustrates our need for trauma.
It is change that we really want.

"When Ferdinand the Unfaithful heard this, he suggested that she should
make the experiment on Ferdinand the Faithful. This, after a while she
did; and after cutting off his head, put it on again, and it healed up, so
that only a red mark was visible around the neck.
'Where did you learn to do that, my child?' asked the king. 'Oh, I
understand it well enough' she replied..."

Ferdinand the Faithful and Ferdinand the Unfaithful
Fairy Tales from Grimm
Wells Gardner Darton and Co 1948

MOTIVATION

Once we have successfully completed the manoeuvre of healing,
we know our core being is adequate for life.

Once we understand this,
we can set our direction and attempt the dance again.
If we can move, we can grow.
If we can grow, we can feel joy.
When we feel joy, we can sense freedom.

This is strength!

Also, we now have a palate of choices.
We now have justice.
We know we can escape from chaos.
We know we can set our direction.
We know we can see the Other in a friend or an enemy.
We know we are looking in a mirror.
We know how to balance the past and the future.
We know how to find love and hate.

This is joy!

"In its full development, the old track was no mean achievement in
surveying and engineering. Road making was not part of its scheme, for
the attitude seems to have been: 'Mother Earth is good enough for you
to walk or ride on, and we will pave a way through the streams, soft places
and ponds; our chief job is to point out the way'.
This the old ley men did magnificently."

Alfred Watkins
The Old Straight Track
Abacus 1974

PALATE

Language of weakness tells us we have nothing,
No resources, no help, no friend, no love.
Language of power gives us permission
to use common sense procedures and ask for help.
There are only two signposts in hell.
One way says, this feels okay. The other way says, this doesn't!

Put onto your palate everything that makes you feel good,
everything that gives you joy, anything and everything that helps you in
any way whatsoever. They are yours to use to comfort yourself.
Put onto your palate every colour of the rainbow,
every smell of the environment that gives you joy,
every sound from the universe that will assist your escape.
Put onto your palate every bit of awareness,
understanding and wisdom that you possess.
Then look at all of it in the mirror and add the reflected image too!
Put onto your palate every memory that you have had, every imprint,
every trauma and every distortion you own.
Circle and spiral into the stream of consciousness
with the strength you now possess.

"You now know a great deal about predicting and avoiding violence, from
the dangers posed by strangers to the brutality inflicted on friends and
family members, from the everyday violence that can touch anyone to the
extraordinary crimes that will touch only a few. With your intuition better
informed, I hope you will have less unwarranted fear of people. I hope
you'll harness and respect you ability to recognise survival signals."

Gavin de Becker
The Gift of Fear
Bloomsbury 1997

PAST

Our past is made up of all of those who succeeded,
all of their best ideas, their best methods, their best beliefs
and their best love to make sure that we are here.

This is not stuff we throw away!

Our past is also made up of all of those who made mistakes, all of their
worst ideas, their worst methods, their worst beliefs and no love at all.

This also is not stuff we throw away!

If we forget the lessons of those who went before us,
we will have to rediscover them for ourselves.
How will we ever have a future
if it is simply made up of repeating the patterns of the past?
How will we ever have a future if we do not learn?
If we never have a future, we will suffer eventual collapse and death.

What of the future then?

"From this it becomes clear that given our diversity no single religion
satisfies all humanity. We can also conclude that we humans can live quite
well without recourse to religious faith."

Dalai Lama
Ancient Wisdom, Modern World
Little, Brown and Co 1999

PERMISSION

Why would we not manage to escape?
Why do we succumb to disease?
Why do we allow chaos, when we don't understand it?
Why do we allow justice to suffer, knowing trauma will result?
Why would we choose pain instead of joy, when escape to freedom is near?
Why don't we change and grow and evolve?
Why do we allow collapse?
Why don't we choose strength and potential instead?
Why would we use language of weakness,
when we could use the language of power?
Why would we forget justice?
Could it be that we have given ourselves permission to do this?
Why would we do that?
What would happen if we allowed ourselves permission
to live and grow strong?
Either way, change and growth or disease must occur.
If we give permission for our direction and motivation
to complete the manoeuvre of escape, we again lose our balance,
which causes distortion, chaos and fear.
This starts the process of healing again.
Life or disease?
Death or healing?

Could permission really be the difference between them?

"From the point of view of ethics it is doubtful whether virtue ever resides
in restrictions imposed from without.
Such so-called virtue is no better than morality which is externally
imposed, herd-induced and often potentially vicious."

Arthur Guirdham
A Theory of Disease
George Allen and Unwin 1957

POTENTIAL

If we are to escape and find wisdom, we must resist the temptation
to name the Other, just so we can hate or love them.

If we are to achieve strength and joy, we must resist the temptation
to blame the Other, just so we can have an enemy or a friend.
To achieve our potential, we must own our own dark side.
We must understand justice, but we must not judge.
We must own our own light side and prevent electric discharge,
which weakens our strength.
We must learn when magnetic energy causes distortion and act accordingly.
Remember that our actions invoke fate.
Note that we do not fully understand it!
Remember that we create the Other
in order to see ourselves more clearly in the mirror.
We need to be kind to ourselves and to the Other.
Wisdom is the key.

"For the person, the difficult and often painful, 'nearly too difficult' as-
signment of becoming what one potentially 'is' includes alternating phases
of illness and healing, of experiencing guilt and redemption, egotism and
sacrifice, and thereby integrating one's separatist or destructive drives into
the 'formal order of the cosmos'."

Edward Whitmont
The Alchemy of Healing
Homeopathic Education Service 1993

PROCESS

Consider a boil.
The initial pain, tenderness, swelling and discolouration,
and then eruption and discharge, indicate a process of healing.
If the reaction can be reabsorbed, it will be.
However, if the manoeuvre is prevented at any point,
disease, even death, can occur.
On all levels of our being, whether disease occurs in our minds,
our spirit, our bodies or our emotions or our language,
it will manifest on all levels of our being.
The wave-like reaction of the process
reflects the distortion through the mirror of trauma.
Our responses can include collapse, disease, death
or healing, life and growth.
The process will vary in subtlety, not in form.
Wisdom dictates that common sense procedures should be followed
and inappropriate treatment avoided.
Justice gives us permission to complete the manoeuvre,
which allows the process of healing to proceed.
Direction is the key.

"No tribal rite has yet been recorded which attempts to keep winter from descending; on the contrary: the rites all prepare the community to endure, together with the rest of Nature, the season of the terrible cold. And in the spring, the rites do not seek to compel Nature to pour forth immediately; on the contrary: the rites dictate the whole people to the cycle of the year, with its hardships and periods of joy, is celebrated and delineated, and represented as continued in the life-round of the human group."

Joseph Campbell
The Hero with a Thousand Faces
Abacus 1975

RED

Red is a powerful colour, encompassing an intense energy spectrum.

Red has a vibration that facilitates strength.
It focuses motivation and enables potential.
It is vigorous and has direction.
Thus survival grasps at this energy of permission.
This vigour is experienced as growth, releasing energy and freedom,
which invigorates awareness.
This energy is full of electric and magnetic energy,
letting us glimpse through the mirror into the universe.
Thus strength is a balance to chaos.
It invigorates life, and it facilitates change.
However, it cannot sustain justice.
This intense energy obscures subtlety.
It obscures focus.
It enables distortion to lead us back into the mirror.
Red energy is thus used to power focal points of momentary clarity,
allowing strength to leap into wisdom through permission.

"... the alder is called Ro-eim ... 'that which reddens the face'; from which
it may be deduced that the 'crimson-stained heroes' of the Welsh Triads,
who were sacred kings, were connected to Bran's alder cult. One reason
for the alders' sanctity is that when it is felled the wood, at first white,
seems to bleed crimson, as though it were a man."

Robert Graves
The White Goddess
Faber and Faber 1975

SPINNING

Next time you are in chaos, sit still and just listen.
Can you sense the spinning?
When you manage to catch your breath, can you hear the spinning?
As your eyes focus, this is balance!

Note how fleeting the sensation is.
Note how soon the spinning turns into white noise and chaos returns.
However, once glimpsed, it fascinates.
Once sensed, it can be imagined and talked about.
What does it mean?
No one knows, but descriptions of it exist from the earliest times.
Today, mystics still try and understand it.

We do not understand the universe, but we think we do.
This makes us dangerous.
When we misjudge our environment,
we must not assume the universe is wrong.
It is most likely us that is wrong!

It is our fate to understand this eventually.

"I tried to breathe, but my breath would not come ... I felt myself rush bodily out of myself and out and out and out and all the time bodily in the wind. I went out swiftly, all of myself, and I knew I was dead and that it had all been a mistake to think you had just died. Then I floated, and instead of going on I felt myself slide back. I breathed and I was back."

Ernest Hemingway
A Farewell to Arms

SPIRAL

To avoid weak ideas, it is important to base our understanding
and our decisions within the spiral of illumination.

Our equations should consider the stream of consciousness.
Each circle of illumination is a discrete point in this stream of consciousness.
All of these points taken together form the universe.
All the spirals contain all the circles, spinning around, forming all there is.

Language of power leads to strong ideas.
For us to understand this larger picture,
we must include everything in our equations.
We must also include the reflections of our equations in the mirror.
These images must reverse to become manifest.
This manifestation of wisdom must be understood
as just part of the dance of life and death.

"The aimlessness, alienation, anomie and violence that characterises so
much of modern life seems to indicate that now they are not deliberately
creating a faith in 'god' or anything else – it matters little what – many
people are falling into despair."

Karen Armstrong
A History of God
Mandarin 1997

STRENGTH

To achieve strength,
we have to know who we are and what we have been.
We can then project our survival into the future.
We must allow ourselves permission to reach for freedom.
We need to understand our potential.
We have to evolve, accept our fate and meet the universe.

This manoeuvre can only be achieved successfully if we understand
everything that we have been, all that we are and all that we can be.
Also, we need to know what we want, what we have wanted and what
we might want. Then we need to study our reflection in the mirror.
This image must reverse to become manifest.

The past and the future dance in an endless stream of consciousness
that connects life and death.
Motivation and permission combine, allowing us to evolve.
Escape becomes possible, circling into freedom.

"Wheat is not quite as adaptable as man, who exceeds all other species in the
range of environments in which he can survive ... but it has spread out over
the world more dramatically, invaded more new habitats, multiplied faster and
evolved more rapidly without extinction than any other known organism. It
now covers more than 600 million acres of the surface of the planet."

Felipe Fernandez Armesto
Civilisations
Macmillan 2000

SURVIVAL

Life is always set towards achieving its potential.
Healing is set deep in our genus species.
However, our direction is not!

If distortion and disease constantly prevent balance,
trauma may result in collapse and death.
Healing may seem too hard or too painful,
so we need the strength to complete the manoeuvre of escape.
We need permission to experience joy.
If we cannot approach joy, why should we even bother?

The language of power implies permission.
The language of weakness denies it.

Magnetic attraction and electric repulsion reverse through the mirror,
so fast our spinning thoughts can enter the circle of illumination.
This triggers the dance of life and death on and on.

"Athene's cry struck panic into the Ithacans, who let their weapons go, in
their terror at the goddesses voice. The arms all fell to earth, and the men
turned citywards, intent on their own salvation. The indomitable Odysseus
raised a terrible war cry, gathered himself together and pounced on them
like a swooping eagle. But at this moment Zeus let fly a flaming bolt,
which fell in front of the bright eyed daughter of that formidable sire.
Athene called out at once to Odysseus by his royal titles, commanding
him to hold off his hand and bring this civil strife to a finish, for fear of
offending the ever watchful Zeus."

Homer
The Odyssey
Penguin 1966

TRAUMA

As we encounter forces current in the universe,
we name them but we do not understand them.

As we experience forces current in the universe,
we meet disease, which triggers a response from us.
We do not understand these forces, or our own response to them.
Thus, we enter chaos and we must seek balance and wisdom to escape.
We conjure words to describe our environment,
but our words are only words.
We invent words that try and force order onto existence,
but we cannot understand.
We appeal to justice, as if existence also speaks our words,
has our ideas, but it does not understand us.

We are just reflections in the mirror,
perceived dimly by the enormous forces playing about above our heads.
All we see through the mirror is ourselves peering back.
Neither of us understands the Other.

Electric and magnetic energy dance all around us.

"Crushed against a pillar, unable to move in the dense mass, he pressed
his hands over his ears. He could not shut out those shrieks! When
would they end? What in the name of the god of mercy were they doing?
Tearing her piecemeal? Yes, and worse than that. And still the shrieks rang
on, and still the great Christ looked down on Philammon with that calm,
intolerable eye, and would not turn away."

Charles Kingsley
Hypatia
Macmillan 1889

UNDERSTAND

We only use ten percent of our consciousness.
Worms crawling in the mud with other worms.
Worms will no doubt be still around when we are gone.

We started with only appetite to satisfy, which gave us joy.
We do not know how we will end.
We do understand that ultimately we must end.
What continues on is up to the universe, not to us!

We pursue joy now at the expense of our appetites,
which we know change and can betray us.
We pursue life because we are life.
We pursue justice, because it prevents trauma.
We grow strong and proliferate, peeking into every crack and cranny
in our desperate urge to satisfy our appetites.

But we do not really know what they are!

"Once consciousness was established, there was no going back, for individuals less well endowed would be at a disadvantage. Similarly, those with a slight edge would be further favoured. An arms race would ensue, driving the process ever onward, boosting intelligence and sharpening self awareness. As the inner eye became ever more observant, inexorably there would emerge a real sense of self, a reflective consciousness, an inner I."

Richard Leakey
The Origin of Humankind
Phoenix 1995

UNIVERSE

The universe is something beyond our knowledge.

To approach it, we need strength and balance.
Our motivation must allow us to manoeuvre.
We must have our own permission to proceed.
Without wisdom, we are lost.

Survival in this environment has always been difficult.
But we have always been here.
The past bears our record, but the future may forget us.
The universe may refashion life in another species.
We have no written guarantee for evolution in this form.
We have no guarantee of survival in any form!

The spinning of the stream of consciousness
may or may not be our permanent home, but it may be our only home.
Escape or extinction is always possible.
Justice is our own creation.

See how far we are from our potential?

"Their less splendid but substantial and permanent reputation is based on their persistent enunciation of a theory of universal development, which true and farsighted adepts well perceived, had an equal application to the triune man as to those metals which in their conception had also a triune nature."

Arthur Waite
Alchemists through the Ages
Rudolph Steiner 1970

WISDOM

Black, white and red are primal ancestral colours
from the very roots of our beginnings.
The number *three* is also in our origin.
Red, white and black combine in infinite and intricate subtlety
in the dance of life and death.
Wisdom requires that all information be gathered
into a circle of illumination, and set in place in
the stream of consciousness so we become strong in its service.
Balance must be achieved, as strength competes with fate.
Everything that exists and everything that does not exist
must be glimpsed through the mirror.
We need to come to grips with our true nature
and stop fooling ourselves that distortion is truth.
We do not set the universe.
It exists without us.
We do not set the patterns of nature.
They were there before us.
We do not understand anything really,
as our subjective realities must always fall short of the environment.
All we really have left is our potential for change and growth.

" 'Justice!'
'Ah, fairest wisdom, don't mention that horrid word out of the lecture
room. In theory it is all very well; but in poor imperfect, earthly practice,
a governor must be content with doing very much what comes to hand.
In abstract justice, now, I ought to nail up Cyril, deacons, district visitors,
and all, in a row on the sand hills outside. That is simple enough; but, like
a great many simple and excellent things, impossible.' "

Charles Kingsley
Hypatia
Macmillan 1889

"Again, the spell, so to speak, by aid of which man escapes from death, triumphs over it, consists in power derived from knowing the whole of its cause. That is, the secrets of death must be plumbed and accurately understood before the soul can triumph."

Lewis Spence
The Mysteries of Britain
Senate 1994

THE LOST BLACK BOOK OF HEALING

For my mother.

Wisdom.
"Were you always wise?
You were the wisest person I ever met.
Life is wise and you embodied this.
The past lived within you.
It formed you.
We are your future."

January 2002

In order to achieve wisdom,
we need to know our place in existence and gain awareness.
This will allow us to accept our destiny with equanimity.
The process of life and death will lead to wisdom through understanding.
This process is part of our fate and it allows us to fulfil our potential.

The only thing that can prevent this process is the universe.

AWARENESS

For aeons, we have sought awareness.
We study and sacrifice, scrimp and save,
spend and bankrupt ourselves in its pursuit.

We criticise Others who are not aware.
We think we are.
We question Others who do not question, believing that we do.
We enter competitions to prove our knowledge,
believing this to be equivalent.
We grasp at knowledge, we want to be near people
who have knowledge, thinking that it will make us wise.

But a small child has awareness, so do the lilies in the field.
All life has awareness, but we judge it condescendingly,
comparing our awareness to our bank balance
or our material possessions, as if this proves anything!

The small child and the lilies and all life laugh at us, but they keep it hidden.
They are afraid of our reaction otherwise.

"Gusts of laughter the Moon stir
That her Bassarids now bed
With the unnoble usurer,
While an ignorant pale priest
Rides the beast with a man's head
To her long-omitted feast."

Robert Graves
The White Goddess
Faber and Faber 1975

BALANCE

The only constant in the universe is change.
We can only achieve balance momentarily, before the circle moves us on.
Stasis is death, so we must plunge back into the maelstrom,
as fate dictates.

How do we find direction?
What can we do with this knowledge?
White energy is used to form a focal point.
Red energy is used to power focal points.
Black energy is used to visualise existence.

We have a circle of illumination forming multiple points
in the spiral of the stream of consciousness,
like white pebbles showing the path through a forest.
All these points taken together form our environment.
Balance points are fulcrums or focal points,
like stepping-stones across a lake.
We must give ourselves permission to manoeuvre, to face our potential.
We must seek direction and contentment as we begin to dance and sing.

Electric and magnetic energy dances around the scene.

"I am old, I am young, I am Gwion,
Universal, I am gifted with a perceiving spirit.
I am a bard, I do not vouchsafe my secrets to slaves.
I am a guide, I am a judge ..."

John Matthews
Taliesin, The Riddle Song
Aquarian 1999

BLACK

Black incorporates all colours, but it does not reflect them.
It obscures them.

Black has a vibration that calms life.
It enhances complexity and enables depth.
It is profound, dense and wonderful.
Thus wisdom swells out of the magnitude of experience.
This experience is experienced as reflective.
It releases knowledge and awareness.
This fuels destiny.
Thus profundity generates electric and magnetic energy.
This mirrors truth.
Thus, black energy is a balance to disease.
It is enriching and allows contentment, which can lead to justice.
But it cannot sustain life.
This deep energy blankets growth.
It obscures change.
It cannot maintain the process which is essential to life.
Black energy is thus used to form a view of existence based on calmness,
allowing wisdom to glimpse the universe.

"In the court of weapons
They called me a coward:
I defended my honour,
Fought, fed the eagles.
My sword bears witness,
Put to the war test:
But I don't care to boast
Bloodshed's not my business."

Eyrbyggja Saga
Penguin 1989

CIRCLE

The circle of life and death spins the magnetic and electric energy
that creates the universe.
Each circle forms part of a spiral of existence
in the stream of consciousness.
Dancing and singing, we see our footsteps in the environment.
We study our reflection in the mirror.
We try to perceive the structure of the whole.
Nothing can be left out.
Three hundred and sixty degrees of all there is,
plus its reflection in the mirror.
This now becomes our playground of experience.
We circle round and round.
We move along the spiral pathways.
We find our direction as we manoeuvre.
We perfect our process.
As our truth continually evolves, we grow into awareness.
Distortion causes trauma, which we can use to promote growth.
Balance causes stasis, which we use to focus our understanding.
Confusion is a healthy state.
Its presence proves our feet upon the path.
Permission to proceed with wisdom is all we need now.

"This is the excellent foppery of the world, that when we are sick in
fortune, often the surfeit of our own behaviour, we make guilty of
our disasters the sun, the moon, and the stars; as if we were villains by
necessity, fools by heavenly compulsion, knaves, thieves, drunkards, liars,
and adulterers by an enforced obedience of planetary influence ..."

William Shakespeare
King Lear

COMMON SENSE PROCEDURES

Find at least three people you can communicate and confide in
for support during the process of existence.
This is called a three-legged stool.
Extend this basic structure to include Others
who can teach you about your destiny.
Practice balance and contentment.
Help your body, your mind and your emotions to achieve strength.
Do everything you can to understand your destiny.
Do everything you can to become aware of your footsteps,
because they invoke fate.
Look at yourself clearly in the mirror
and give yourself permission to realise your potential.
Stop using language of defeat.
Don't use inappropriate treatment.
Get off the corkscrew of the hierarchy.
Don't be a perpetrator or a scapegoat.
Practice dancing and singing.
Distinguish awareness, knowledge, confusion, understanding and wisdom.
Study justice. Practice spinning.
Understand that life and death mirror each other.
Balance love and hate.
Balance past and future.
Grow out of friends and enemies.
Study electric and magnetic states.

"There is, in the interior of man, nothing morbid that is curable, and no visible
morbid alteration that is curable which does not make itself known to the
accurately observing physician by means of morbid signs and symptoms."

Samuel Hahnemann
Aphorism 14, The Organon of Medicine

CONFUSION

Complicated issues arouse many different points of view,
all competing together, all intruding into all discussions.

Confusion is consciousness changing.

Hope springs out of confusion as fixed positions change.
Stasis is the death of wisdom.
Change is the only constant in the universe.
Confusion is consciousness growing.

Truth changes with each new fact.
Our palate of knowledge grows.
The more we know, the more we understand.
Confusion is consciousness evolving.

It moves us towards our potential.
The more we know, the more we follow the process.
Confusion is consciousness dancing and singing with existence.
As we move around our environment, the more we find wisdom.
Confusion is consciousness circling and spiralling
along the stream of life and death.

Electric and magnetic energy flickers around the scene.

"The pond is cradled by the mountain,
The superior man feels calm and chivalrous.
Success
If you keep to your course
And remain receptive to others."

Sam Reifler
I Ching, Hexagram 31
Bantam 1981

CONTENTMENT

We will learn to balance all our balance points, eventually.
We can grow and thrive with a full palate.
Trauma can be understood.
Disease can turn to healing.
Common sense procedures can stabilise chaos.
This is strength!
This is life!
This is love!
This is wisdom!
Nothing stays the same. The only constant is change.
We must enter the maelstrom again.
But we may just know how to fly.
We may know how to dance and sing our path to our destiny.
We may know how to recognise our footsteps.
We may just know how to manoeuvre out of trauma.
We may know how to use the process to avoid disease.
We may know how to understand the mirror.
We know how to become aware of our direction.
We know how to use balance to move around our environment.
We know how to use language of wisdom to grow strong.
We know how to avoid language of defeat.
We may know how to balance the past and the future.
We know how to use language of wisdom to act differently.
We may know how to evolve and grow in the spinning universe.
Life or death?
Friend or enemy?
But what do we all want?

"Next, when you are describing a shape, or sound, or tint
Don't state the matter plainly but put it in a hint;
And learn to look at all things with a sort of mental squint."

Lewis Carroll
Poeta Fit, Non Nascitur 1860-1863

DANCING

Now we understand how to manoeuvre
through the process of life and death, we can set our footsteps.
This is our dance of destiny.

Now we can dance, we can circle and spiral around the universe.
This is our present, our strength, our potential and our fate.
Every action evokes an equal and opposite reaction.
Does the universe talk back to us or only echo our actions?
If we copy existence, will it notice that we are doing so?
If we make our own pattern, will the universe see us?
If we invent a hierarchy, we can order existence to obey us.
Can't we?
If we use our strength and our knowledge,
we can make life do as we say.
Can't we?
See how fear feeds distortion, which causes trauma,
which causes disease, which causes fear?
On and on in an endless dance?
On and on until we give ourselves permission
to stop and find a new direction?

"Well, you can knock me down, step in my face,
Slander my name all over the place,
Burn my house, steal my car,
Drink my liquor from my old fruit jar;
But don't you step on my blue suede shoes."

Carl Lee Perkins
Blue Suede Shoes, 1956

DEATH

Death is part of life.
We are finite and infinite creatures.

We must understand our true nature,
or our equations will be inadequate for our survival.
Knowing this prevents trauma and disease.

We can set the direction of our core being.
We can give ourselves permission to dance and sing
as we study ourselves in the mirror.
We can heal our motivation and go forward into the future.
This is Wisdom!

Our potential is set deep in our genus species.
We will evolve as long as we can grow and thrive.
Its not as if we really have to do anything else to do.
We seek joy and contentment.
We seek truth and justice.
We want freedom.
We wait for wisdom.

This is what the lilies in the field do to express perfection
as they decorate our environment.

"Too late, my time has come,
Sends shivers down my spine, body's aching all the time,
Goodbye, everybody, I've got to go,
Gotta leave you all behind and face the truth,
Mama, ooh, I don't want to die,
I sometimes wish I'd never been born at all."

Freddie Mercury and Queen
Bohemian Rhapsody, 1975

DESTINY

Where are we all going?
What do we all want?
What is our purpose?
Where will it all end?

Life has evolved with the universe.
We have emerged from chaos.
We have always been here, first in primitive form; now we are complex.
Will we become more complex or will we find simplicity?
When we understand existence, will we find contentment?
When we can dance and sing, will we find joy?
When we peer into the mirror, what potential do we see?
Will we go forward into the future with direction?
Can we balance ourselves?
Can we set our motivation to ensure our survival?
Can we love the Other as well as hate them?
Will we hate hierarchy
because it causes trauma, isolation, fear and disease?
Or do we see through it all and collapse back into chaos
because it is all too difficult and distorted?

"Many times I've been alone,
And many times I've cried,
Anyway, you'll never know how many times I've tried,
But still they lead me back to the long and winding road."

John Lennon and Paul McCartney
The Long and Winding Road, 1970

DIRECTION

In order to complete a manoeuvre, we need direction.

In an energy landscape, we can do any magic manoeuvre we can think of
(and many we can't!)
In the environment of the imagination, we can be everywhere at once.
Do we go up or down, side-to-side, front to back, inside out, outside in?
Do we circle and spiral towards the past or the future?
Or do we stand still?
Do we dance and sing into infinity or into the finite?
Do we grow large or become very small?
We can move towards or move away, or do both.
Why would we do any of this?
We could do anything!
We could do nothing!
All of these are directions.
They are all available to us.
There are only two signposts in hell.
One says, this feels okay.
The other one says, this doesn't!
One way leads to death.
The other leads to life!

"The whole book has been dominated by the idea of chance, by the
astronomically long odds against the spontaneous arising of order,
complexity and apparent design. We have sought a way of taming chance,
of drawing its fangs. 'Untamed chance', pure, naked chance, means
ordered design springing into existence from nothing, in a single leap."

The Blind Watchmaker
Richard Dawkins
Penguin 1991

DISEASE

Disease is observable as a shockwave rippling out.
This causes a secondary reaction from life
as all levels of existence experience distortion.
This is movement!
Stasis is death!
Balance is only ever momentary.
Change is the only constant in the universe.
For every action there is an equal and opposite reaction.
Seen through the mirror,
disease is the reflected image of the trauma that caused it.
Seen through the mirror,
healing is the reflected image of the disease that caused it.
The dance simply reverses, exact and step for step.
It all depends upon our direction.
Seen through the mirror, dancing and singing are the reflected image
of the original drama of life and death emerging from original chaos.
Disease takes many forms, and the reaction of life in response is equally complex.
Life takes many forms, and the reaction of disease in response is just as varied.

But the patterns match in the mirror.

"I am no vexed courier,
I do not avenge what offends me,
I laugh no laugh
Under the worms.
My knee is outstretched
In the earthen house,
With an iron chain,
Around my knees.

J T Koch
Taliesin
The Goddodin of Aneirin
University of Wales Press 1997

DISTORTION

Distorted functioning on any level can quickly lead to awareness.
Subtle changes will eventually be as illuminating as major changes.
Distortion of out-moded states is wonderful news in some cases.
In others, it is worrying.
Major changes can be as subtle as minor fluctuations.
This is a difficult time!
We have to change and grow if we are to thrive.
We have to give ourselves permission to balance.
We have to allow understanding. We have to permit justice.
We have to succumb to confusion.
We must understand the separation of the hierarchy.
We must feel the fear of the perpetrator and of the scapegoat.
Things still seem distorted.
We must touch our enemy and our friend in the mirror.
We need to know our direction.
We must clearly perceive the distortion of the mirror.
We must use common sense procedures.
We must avoid inappropriate treatment.
We must set our clock of fate as we go dancing and singing through the universe.
Things still seem chaotic.
We must learn the language of wisdom.
Mortal or immortal beings, we face the future.

"We're so glad to see so many of you lovely people here tonight, and we
would especially like to welcome all the representatives of Illinois's law
enforcement community who have chosen to join us here in the Palace Hotel
Ballroom at this time. We do sincerely hope you all enjoy the show, and please
remember people, that no matter who you are and what you do to live, thrive
and survive, there are still some things that make us all the same ..."

B Berns, S Burke and J Wexler
Everybody Needs Somebody to Love, 1964

ELECTRIC

Electric energy is overwhelming.
It is either there or it is not there.
Magnetic energy shimmers in the aftermath.
Being overwhelmed causes trauma and increases awareness.
Never being overwhelmed can also cause trauma.
The presence or absence of electric energy causes distortion.
Both states enable change, growth or death.
This drama is instrumental to our knowledge.
Its very nature demonstrates ideas of destiny.
Its effect on us is profound and of vital importance to our being.
It is neither our servant nor our master.
Such thinking is the product of the hierarchy.
Such equations are the product of distortion.
Such beliefs are formed by confusion, which forces us to become
either a perpetrator or a scapegoat to disguise our fear.
This is not strength!
This is not wisdom!
If this is our future, our motivation will fail, our direction will fade
and we will become our own enemy, our own disease.
Balance alternates with chaos in the dance of life and death.
Electric and magnetic energy flickers around the scene.
We still perceive dimly through the mirror.

"Restlessness, anxiety and anguish, sometimes more particularly in the chest, internal anguish, violent agitation, timidity. Fear on the approach of a storm. Ill humour. Involuntary laughter. Furor. Loss of consciousness, insensibility, foolish actions, haggard eyes. Errors in the appreciation of time, loss of memory."

Robin Murphy
Electricitas
Lotus Materia Medica 1995

ENEMY

The enemy is different from the Other.
The Other is just different from us, and only becomes an enemy
when we see our own distorted image in the mirror. Things may be real
or imagined, but they will trigger an automatic reaction from us.
Initially, we have a trauma that we need to process.
So we look in the mirror and project our disease onto an Other.
We identify our scapegoat through magnetic attraction
triggered by the similarity between the Other and ourselves.
This can then be perceived as the origin of the original trauma.
The circle turns.
Electric energy shimmers around the scene as we project our distortion
out into the environment.
Thus we become our own enemy and the enemy of Others.
Reflected back through the mirror, our actions become our fate.
By allowing ourselves permission to distort the image of an Other,
we express our own trauma and indulge in cruelty to ease our fear.
This is an aggressive act.
This is the first step in the construction of a hierarchy.
This is a building block of disease.
This is the cornerstone of death.

"Look at yourself in the mirror and make that change."
Michael Jackson

"The three now threatened to set fire to the house if the landlord did
not give them a large sum of money, and the poor man was compelled to
give them all he could scrape together, with which they went away. But
although they had enough to last them their lifetime, each would rather
have had his own hand, heart or eyes than all the money in the world."
The Three Army Surgeons
Fairy Tales from Grimm
Wells Gardener, Darton and Co 1948

ENVIRONMENT

What we believe forms our environment.
What we believe sets our existence!
What we think dictates what we get.
What we think dictates our understanding!
What we say dictates what we believe.
What we say we think we believe!
To harmonise our life,
we need to understand the reversal through the mirror.
We must harmonise our energy before we can find balance,
before we can see a focus, before we can use a fulcrum,
before we can make any change.
If we do not balance, we will spiral into distortion, chaos and disease.
We experience this as trauma.
If we do not balance, we spread our trauma and our chaos
and our distortion out into the universe,
forcing an equal and opposite reaction from it.
Then we turn around and see the distorted image of the Other
in the mirror and we displace our fear onto them.
Thus we create a hierarchy and take up our position within it.
Perpetrator or scapegoat, friend or enemy,
we turn fear and chaos into trauma.
We force electric and magnetic energy to discharge into our environment.
Then we blame our scapegoat and begin to look for enemies.
Our dance of life and death spins on and on into an uncertain future.

"He gave her his town house and his racing horses,
Each meal she ate was a dozen courses,
Had a million dollars worth of nickels and dimes,
She sat around and counted them all a million times."

Cab Calloway and Irving Mills
Minnie the Moocher, 1932

EXISTENCE

So we are here!
We are all here!
This is all there is!
That's it!
We are clinging to a rock hurtling through space screaming our heads off!
Great!
All those multitudinous individuals, spinning through the universe,
All seeking joy, love, hate.
All those multitudinous individuals dancing and singing.
All reflected in the mirror, all are Others.
We are alone!
As we circle and spiral around this shocking scene,
electric and magnetic energy flickers all around.
This is fear, but it will become understanding.
This is hate, but it will become love.
This is disease, but it strengthens life.
This is ignorance, but it will become awareness.
We want truth, justice, wisdom.
And we will do anything to get it,
even if it means using the hierarchy to cause trauma to Others.
Better them than us!
And we will do it, even if it means understanding wisdom. Even if it means
dismantling the hierarchy and accepting our oneness with the Other.
Better together than alone!

"Day after day, alone on the hill,
The man with the foolish grin is keeping perfectly still,
But nobody wants to know him,
They can see that he's just a fool,
And he never gives an answer –
But the fool on the hill sees the sun going down
And the eyes in his head see the world spinning 'round."

John Lennon and Paul McCartney
The Fool on the Hill, 1967

FATE

Once we start to become aware of fate,
we must assume responsibility for our actions!
Once we notice our footsteps,
we can retrace the path that brought us here.
We are our own actions!
Once we see the Other in the mirror,
we can see that they are our exact opposite, and strangely similar.
We are our Other!
Once we hear our own singing, we understand that we mask
Other singers, Other songs.
We are not alone!
Once we move our feet and dance, we can see
Other's footsteps in the earth.
We are not alone!

Whatever our beliefs, our actions, our words, our dance of life and death
will create and define us, the society around us and the political and
religious structures that result.
It all depends upon our permission.

We have reached the mirror.
It is a start!

"You spoiled the best years of your life,
You took them all in vain,
Now you think that you're forgiven,
But you can't be born again.
And you say why?"

Annie Lennox and Dave Stewart
Don't Ask Me Why, 1989

FEAR

Fear has enormous power over us.
We have relied on it to keep us safe in a dangerous world.
We have always relied on fear to warn us of danger.
Today we need it to teach us the sound of the universe.
Fear creates an instinctual reaction in us.
We look around for an enemy.
When we find one, we magnetically alter fear by distorting the mirror.
We create a hierarchy.
We gain a position in relation to fear.
We have an Other.
Its not me, it's you!
We are safe?
Fear causes trauma, causing us to become aware.
Fear allows us to perceive an enemy and eject our trauma.
Its not me, it's you!
Are we safe?
Fear causes confusion.
It causes the present to dance with the past and the future.
Fear causes trauma and disease, as we struggle to become aware.
Fear causes justice, as we fight for life.
Fear causes wisdom, as we struggle to understand.
Fear causes change and growth and survival.
Fear causes the hierarchy.
Its not me, it's you!
We are definitely not safe!
Fear has a magnetic attraction.
It satisfies our voyeuristic fascination.

"Showed me different shapes and colours, showed me many different roads,
Gave me very clear instructions, when I was in the dark night of the soul."

Van Morrison
Tore Down A La Rimbaud, 1984

FRIEND

A friend is different from the Other.
We can manoeuvre around the Other as a friend or as an enemy.
We can love or hate them.
We can practice our perpetrator and our scapegoat.
We can practice our dancing and singing.
We can learn to manoeuvre around our environment.
As we move, we create a hierarchy.
We circle and spiral around our reflections in the mirror.
Past, present and future spin around us.
Electric and magnetic energy flickers around the scene.
Confusion and awareness challenge knowledge and truth.
Trauma and disease emerge.
Language of wisdom becomes language of defeat.
Language of past distorts the language of the future.
Concepts of justice arise.
This triggers the process of the dance of life and death.
Healing and disease reflect each other.
Each reaction is an equal and opposite reflection of consciousness.
It all depends upon our direction.

Can we allow ourselves permission to understand this?

"For you, and such as you, it is still a pleasure to gather bindweed
thoughts and dreams; still a pleasure to gather dreams, these thoughts,
to the airs and pauses and harmonies of considered speech. So by your
acceptance of this book, let me be not only of your fellowship, but of that
little scattered clan to whom wild bees of the spirit come, as secret wings
in the dark, with the sound and breath of forgotten things."

The Avalonians
Patrick Benham
Gothic Image 1993

FUTURE

We glimpse the future brightly through our solar plexus.
Our emotions enmesh us!
We use language of past to discuss it, but language of defeat
will not lead us to our future, which is rooted in the past.
As we look forward, our awareness is distorted by the surface
of the mirror, like a reed stem refracted by a pool of water.
We feel the pull in our minds, but it is language of wisdom
that allows us to do justice to existence.
We feel the pull in our throat, but it is language of past that emerges.

What is false?
What is truth?

We feel the pull in our heart,
but we fail our potential if we cannot balance knowledge and truth.
We feel the pull in our belly,
but we cannot tell if our knowledge is wisdom.

"The road goes ever on and on
Down from the door where it began.
Now far ahead the road has gone,
And I must follow it if I can,
Pursuing it with eager feet,
Until it joins some larger way
Where many paths and errands meet.
And whither then?
I cannot say ..."

J R R Tolkien
The Lord of the Rings
George Allen and Unwin 1969

HATE

Hate is blind, but it can see!
It can see into the stream of consciousness
because it needs to hate the enemy.
The grand scheme of the present suffers distortion,
allowing contentment through trauma caused to Others.

Hate will discover language of wisdom
in order to get permission for justice.
Hate protects life in anticipation.
Spinning out of chaos, awareness sees through the mirror
through the clarity of hate.
Understanding dawns as knowledge and confusion coalesce into wisdom.
Dancing and singing along the stream of consciousness,
hate spirals and circles in and out of the mirror.

Love is always that close!
Sometimes wisdom is dearly bought!
The call to hate or love is very strong.
It will bring the salmon upstream.

Electric and magnetic energy shimmers around the scene.

"It's gilt-edged, glamorous and sleek by design,
You know it's jealous by nature, false and unkind.
It's hard and restrained and it's totally cool,
It touches and it teases as you stumble in the debris."

Annie Lennox and Dave Stewart
Love is a Stranger, 1982

HEALING

Healing is observable as a shockwave rippling out.
This causes a secondary reaction from death
as all layers of existence demonstrate distortion.

This is change!
This is movement!
Balance is only ever momentary!
Chaos is always that close!

As life and death reverse through the mirror,
healing becomes the ability to understand.
As disease and healing reflect each other,
the original trauma resolves like a bruise coming out.
The original trauma is always the reflected image
of the hierarchy we imposed as we separated ourselves from the Other.
This allowed us to define our difference
as we see only the similarity of the Other,
fighting over the scarce resources in our environment.

Fear is always that close!
Justice is born.

"I think I can make it now, the pain has gone,
All of the bad feelings have disappeared.
Here is the rainbow I've been praying for,
It's gonna be a bright, bright, bright sunshiny day."

Johnny Nash
Sunshiny Day, 1972

HIERARCHY

It is the nature of scum to rise to the surface.
It is the nature of elements to separate in a centrifuge.
This is knowledge.
It is the nature of fear to threaten existence.
This is not balance, but it can cause us to find it.
It is the nature of fear to separate us from the Other,
so we can escape from pain.
It is the nature of a perpetrator to cause trauma.
This is cruelty.
It is the nature of the scapegoat to accept distortion,
so it can deflect the truth.
This is language of defeat.
It is the nature of hate and love to create an Other.
This is so we can stare at each Other in the mirror.
Maybe then we can see more clearly?

Distortion unhooks the mind and contentment is lost.
Trauma alters language and our ability to understand.
This unhooks the emotions.
Through the mirror we become the perpetrator and the scapegoat.
We circle and spiral, dancing and singing all awry.
This unhooks the body.

Disease is born!

"Some things in life are bad,
They can really make you mad.
Other things just make you swear and curse.
When you're chewing on life's gristle
Don't grumble, give a whistle,
And this'll help things turn out for the best."

Eric Idle
Always Look on the Bright Side of Life, 1979

INAPPROPRIATE TREATMENT

Matching individual circumstances with appropriate treatment
must give us a better chance to assist the process of healing.
How do we expect to heal if we cannot manoeuvre?
How do we expect to survive unless we develop strength?
We must give ourselves permission to use our palate.
We must apply what we have learnt to ensure our survival.
If we block ourselves, we become our own enemy.
If we deny ourselves, we become our own distortion.
If we hurt ourselves, we become our own disease.
If we drug ourselves, we become our own trauma.
If we cling to the hierarchy, we become our own scapegoat.
If we don't look in the mirror, we become our own perpetrator.
If we love or hate the Other, we fear to face them openly.
If we need a friend or an enemy, we will never find ourselves.

"The age of the patient, his mode of living and diet, his occupation, his
domestic position, his social relations and so forth must next be taken
into consideration, in order to ascertain whether these things have tended
to increase his malady, or in how far they may not favour or hinder the
treatment. In like manner the state of his disposition and mind must be
attended to, to learn whether that presents any obstacle to the treatment,
or required to be directed, encouraged or modified."

Samuel Hahnemann
Aphorism 208, The Organon of Medicine

JUSTICE

Old sins cast long shadows.
Note how completely the shadow shape fits into the environment?
The two are one!
Through the mirror, we can see the distortion in the universe.
Our shadows represent us.
All those multitudinous differences, all allowed?
All those billions of individual shadows, dancing and singing?
All competing for all resources?
All those appetites, seeking to be satisfied?
All seeking life, contentment and joy?
All seeking death, trauma and hate?
Whatever gets you through the night!
Justice is all we have until we find wisdom.
Justice is all we have until we find understanding, fate and destiny.
Whatever gets you through the day!
It is not over till the Fat Lady sings!

"... syphilitic rashes may itch and that prurigo is infectious and is one of the initial stages of leprosy. This boy had a spot on the left thigh to size of a man's thumb. This was distinctly a leper spot. Syph 1000c caused the rash to come out strongly all over the body in patches, the face was one third covered with thick, yellow, scabby eruption. The remedy was continued and the boy got well, wonderfully improved in health, no longer nervous, growing well, sleeping well, appetite good."

Syphylinum, Lotus Materia Medica
Robin Murphy 1995

KNOWLEDGE

Using our palate, we have collected all our knowledge.
All our healing and all our disease.
All our understanding of fate.
All our awareness about our potential.
All our accrued wisdom.
What sort of equations can we make now?
Is it enough?
Are our facts in the right order, the right pattern?
We have many skills, but are they sufficient?
We have lots of knowledge, but is this wisdom?
We become frantic and fear builds, causing distortion in the mirror.
Our palate can only reflect the truth when it reaches all there is.
Three hundred and sixty degrees.
Totality!
This totality then needs to add its own reflection in the mirror
for the manoeuvre to become complete.
But note that people are here now, in the present.
They were also there in the past.
Dancing and singing in imperfection, practising songs and dances
that have pattern in the universe.
We survived through the aeons, proliferating and growing.

We do this in the teeth of chaos!

"The true knowledge obtained for them by the Druid of the Cruithnigh,
at once, was that thrice fifty hornless cows of the plain
be milked in one deep hollow."

John Matthews
The Druid Source Book
Blandford 1997

LANGUAGE OF DEFEAT

Know that language is alive, that it is a tool! It can be used as a tool!
Human language is extraordinarily complex.
Each language contains many different forms of speech within it.
Different forms of speech are used to describe different aspects of life.
We can try out different behaviours,
different strategies, different perceptions.
We can give ourselves permission or we can deny it.
It all depends upon our direction and our motivation.
It all depends on our awareness and understanding.
It all depends upon our knowledge and our wisdom.
It all depends upon our actions and the reflections we elicit from the Other.
It all depends upon our dancing and singing
as we circle and spiral around the universe.
It all depends upon our appetites and on our confusion.

There are only two signposts in hell.
One way says, this feels okay. The other way says, this doesn't!
It all depends upon your direction!
All there is forms and reforms in our environment,
distorted like a reed stem refracted by a pool of water.
It is our fate to understand this eventually!

"Thus began the age of despair.
The roads were tangled.
The winds and the sandstorms dwelt in the husks of cities,
The plains and mountains became our home.
As the old gods lost their power,
We called to the blank sky
Into the cold, dividing gray to the ears of new gods,
The sky is calm, silent, unmoving.
We have yet to hear their answer."

Michael Williams
Canticle of the Dragon Part II, The Complete Krynn Source Book
TSR Inc 1987

LANGUAGE OF FUTURE

We glimpse the future through the mirror, which distorts truth
like a reed stem refracted by a pool of water.
We need strength, permission and wisdom to face the universe.
We need to know the patterns of the past.
We need to face our true nature.
We need to be able to circle and spiral around our environment.
We need to be skilled at dancing and singing.
We need to be wise to meet our destiny.
We need to know fear and choose kindness.
If future conditions are completely different from anything that has
gone before, we need to sing our own song and dance our own dance.
We need to speak our own language to evolve.
Change is the only constant in the universe.
Everything changes but everything also stays the same.
Infinite combinations lead to infinite diversity.
All we need is love.

"Infinite diversity in infinite combination."
Star Trek IDIC
Paramount Pictures

"On a divinatory level, the card of Chronos the Hermit augurs a time of
aloneness or withdrawal from the extraverted activities of life, so that the
wisdom of patience may be acquired. There is an opportunity to build
solid foundations if one is willing to wait. Thus the fool at last arrives at
maturity, having developed a mind and a heart, a firm sense of identity and
finally a deep respect for his own limitations in the great passage of the
round of time."
Juliet Sharman Burke and Liz Green
The Hermit, The Mythic Tarot
Rider 1986

LANGUAGE OF PAST

We glimpse the past through the mirror, which distorts truth
like a reed stem refracted by a pool of water.
We search through the flotsam and jetsam of our ancestors
to find our heart song.
Our emotions enmesh us!
What we find confronts us!
Our true nature is quite a shock!
This is not stuff we throw away! We dig through the earth to touch
what we used to be and to remember the smell and the touch of it.
All those shining ones and their achievements!
All those shining achievements of dangerous parents!
All those revelations of wise elders,
reverberating through our minds from our origins!
Our emotions enmesh us!
Our true nature is still quite a shock!
This is not stuff we throw away!
If we forget the lessons of the past, we are condemned to repeat them.
If we do not see the patterns in these dangerous, wise footsteps,
we will never become aware of our own dance, of our own song.
Our song of the past must honour our ancestors,
but we must go beyond them do this.
We stand on their shoulders, as they wished us to do.
What can we see on our tip-toes?

"I summon today all those between me and those evils,
Against every cruel merciless powers that may oppose my body and soul,
Against incantations of false prophets, against black laws of pagandom,
Against false laws of heretics, against craft of idolatry,
Against spells of women and smiths and wizards,
Against every knowledge that corrupts man's body and soul."

David Adam
The Hymn of St Patrick, The Cry of the Deer
Triangle 1987

LANGUAGE OF WISDOM

Wisdom dictates that all knowledge be gathered onto a palate of
illumination and set in place in the stream of consciousness.
Nothing can be lost!
Everything that exists and everything that does not exist
must be understood despite its refraction in the mirror.
We need to come to grips with our true nature and
stop fooling ourselves that distortion is truth!
For every action there is an equal and opposite reaction.
The universe mirrors our actions as we create our own destiny.
Singing a different song from existence will cause distortion.
Singing the same song as the universe will also cause distortion.
Dancing away from life can only cause trauma.
Dancing the pattern of wisdom can only enhance justice.
Once this is understood, we can begin to allow ourselves
permission to become wise.
Black, white and red are primal ancestral colours in all peoples from the
very roots of their beginnings.
Each colour has a sound.
Each colour has a pattern.
Each colour has an energy.
Each colour has a balance point.
This knowledge allows us to emerge from chaos to blink at the sun.

"Though here at journey's end I lie
In darkness buried deep,
Beyond all towers strong and high,
Beyond all mountains steep,
Above all shadows rides the sun
And stars forever dwell:
I will not say the day is done,
Nor bid the stars farewell."

J R R Tolkien
The Lord of the Rings
George Allen and Unwin 1969

LIFE

In the dance of life and death, both states mirror each other.
Both have equal power over us.
Both states are our destiny.
But life is stronger than death.
Death only leads to extinction, but life proliferates endlessly.
Even in death, life is thinking!

From death, life emerges, spinning through the universe,
the two states entwine to create each other.
Balance is a pivot point between life and death,
between chaos and awareness.
What we understand grows as we evolve.
Knowledge accumulates as we grow.
Wisdom emerges as we understand the process of healing, as we
comprehend existence, as we sense the distortion of the hierarchy.
We see through the mirror like a reed stem refracted by a pool of water.
We must understand the colours of healing
and develop the language to speak our potential.
This is wisdom!
This is contentment!

"On a divinatory level, the card of the Star when it appears in a spear
portends the experience of hope, meaning and faith in the midst of
difficulties. Although the star to can be ambivalent, and can warn against
blind hope without the necessary action to build upon it, the card of the
star is an augury or promise, an altogether welcome experience for the
fool who passed through the collapse of everything which he believed to
be of value in his life."

Juliet Sharman Burke and Liz Green
The Star, The Mythic Tarot
Rider 1986

LOVE

Love is blind but it can see.
It can see into the stream of consciousness
because it needs to protect that which we love.
The grand scheme of the present achieves contentment.

Love will discover the language of wisdom
in order to get permission for justice.
Love protects life in anticipation.

Spinning out of chaos, awareness sees through the clarity of love.
Understanding dawns as knowledge and confusion separate into wisdom.

Dancing and singing along the stream of consciousness,
love spirals and circles in and out of the mirror.

Hate is always that close!

The call to love or hate is very strong.
It will bring the salmon upstream.
Electric and magnetic energy flickers around the scene.
Sometimes, wisdom is dearly bought!

"Please don't ask what's on my mind
I'm a little mixed up but I'm feeling fine
When I'm near that girl that I love the best
My heart beats so that it scares me to death!
I'm in love!
I'm all shook up!"

Otis Blackwell and Elvis Presley
All Shook Up, 1957

MAGNETIC

Magnetic energy can appear as a friend.
It can be soft and powerful. It is often disguised or subtle.
We suffer distortion in its presence, just as we distort it for our own ends.
Its very nature causes us to change.
Its absence causes trauma and confusion.
Its absence can damage motivation
and lead to the process of healing or disease.
Its effect on us is profound,
but obscured in ways that are of vital importance to our nature.
Its effect on us is electric, but hidden in ways that are vital to our truth.
We are attracted and repelled by magnetic energy like bees to flowers.
Electric energy discharges all around us.
These two forces cause the universe to circle and spiral to form existence.
These two forces cause us to move and grow and change.
These two forces trigger awareness and understanding
as we use our strength to grasp at life.
These two forces trigger distortion, trauma and disease
as we struggle to avoid death.
These two forces are perceived dimly
as we sense their presence in the faces of Others.
Seen through the mirror, they appear refracted
like a reed stem in a pool of water.

"Peevish and inclination to weep with shivering. Mildness, submission.
Indolence when seated, as if power of moving were lost. Speaking loud
while quite alone and engaged in business. Irresolution, followed by
prompt execution after a resolution has been once formed."

Magnetis Poli Ambo
Lotus Materia Medica
Robin Murphy 1995

MIRROR

Magnetic forces join us to our reflected image.
The reflected image is our Other.
As we separate from the Other, electric energy discharges all around.
Fear of discharge or the desire of it keeps us glued into ways of being,
ways of understanding, ways of confusion, ways of language.
We assess our performance by studying the reflections in the mirror,
in the Other.
Love of discharge, or the fear of it, keeps us stuck into ways of being,
ways of understanding, ways of distortion, ways of language.
We assess our performance by studying the reactions in the mirror,
in the Other.
The Other is anyone who is different from us, but they are also familiar.
It is the similarity that fascinates.
We learn so much from this comparison.
We learn to love and hate.
We learn to live or die.
We learn the process of healing and disease.
We learn to understand cruelty and kindness.
We learn how to manoeuvre around existence.
We learn dancing and singing, spinning around the universe.
We learn that our footsteps cause a spiral, which creates a hierarchy,
which creates distortion and disease.
We learn that we are the Other.
Together we are whole.

"Loneliness was tough, the toughest role you ever played
Hollywood created a superstar, and pain was the price you paid."

Elton John and Bernie Taupin
Candle in the Wind, 1973

PAST

We glimpse the past darkly through our solar plexus.
Our emotions enmesh us!

We use language of defeat to discuss the past,
but language of past will not lead us to our destiny, which is in the future.
As we look back, our understanding is distorted by the surface
of the mirror like a reed stem refracted by a pool of water.

We feel the pull in our belly, we think our knowledge is wisdom,
but it is weakness to create such poor equations.
We feel the pull in our heart,
but it is existence we compromise by our short sight.
We feel the pull in our throat, but it is weakness to deny our process, not
knowing what is false and what is truth.
We feel the pull in our minds,
but it is language of wisdom that will allow us justice.

We need wisdom to know the difference between knowledge and awareness.

"I heard the news today, oh boy,
Four thousand holes in Blackburn, Lancashire.
And though the holes we rather small,
They had to count them all.
Now they know how many holes it takes to fill the Albert Hall."

John Lennon and Paul McCartney
A Day in the Life, 1967

PERMISSION

Could it be that we give ourselves permission to live or die,
to heal or suffer disease?

Could it be that we have given ourselves permission to become ill?
Could it be that we have to allow ourselves to grow and thrive?

Why would we choose pain instead of joy?
Why do we allow justice to suffer, knowing that trauma will result?
Why don't we prevent damage to our environment?
Why do we love?
Why do we need a friend or an enemy?
Why do we need to be a perpetrator or a scapegoat?
Why would we do any of these things?

What happens if we allow ourselves contentment?
What happens if we allow ourselves permission
to live and grow and thrive?

What permission do we give to ourselves?
What permission do we allow to Others?

"Because I was afraid to speak when I was just a lad,
Me father gave me nose a tweak and told me I was bad.
But then one day I learned a word that saved me aching nose,
The biggest word you ever heard, and this is how it goes ..."

Richard M Sherman and Robert B Sherman
Supercalifragilisticexpialidocious, 1963

PERPETRATOR

If we do not understand the Other,
they will threaten us with their difference and their similarity.

While we circle and spiral around the hierarchy,
the Other competes with us for resources.
Viewed from this position, the Other is either above us or below us,
challenging our environment.
When we see the Other in the mirror,
they are our own distorted image.
When we love or hate the Other,
we are only reacting to our own appetite for a friend or an enemy.
While we fear the Other, we are slaves to distortion and fear.

As long as we give ourselves permission,
we can glare at the Other to forgive ourselves.
As long as we live in the hierarchy,
we can react to the Other to explain ourselves.
As long as we are diseased,
we can speak of the Other to justify ourselves.
As long as we are traumatised,
we can blame the Other as we exonerate ourselves.
As long as we believe we are alone,
we can fear the Other because they are separate from us.

Coming together is always that close.

"He's got the whole world in his hands;
He's got the night and day in his hands;
He's got the spring and fall in his hands;
He's got the whole world in his hands."

He's Got the Whole World in His Hands
Dorsey Brothers Music 1981

POTENTIAL

It is our potential to understand the universe.
It is our potential to evolve and find wisdom.
It is our potential to balance life and death.
It is our potential to reject cruelty and embrace kindness.
It is our potential to redress trauma and ease disease.
It is our potential to love our environment.
It is our potential to heal the Other, only to find we have healed ourselves.
It is our potential to allow the perpetrator and scapegoat
to touch in the mirror.
It is our potential to balance the past, present and future.
It is our potential to become aware of existence.
It is our potential to become strong, to change and to evolve.
It is our potential to remember the baby in the bathwater.
It is our potential to understand fate.
It is our potential to own our dark side.
It is our potential to safely earth trauma and to protect life.

"The death referred to is not the death of the body, since for such a death
there is no need of resurrection. For if there is a soul, and moreover an
immortal soul, it can dispense with a resurrection of the body ... the death
which might occur even during life, that is to say, of the death of that
"tyrant" from whom proceeds our slavery in this life ..."

G I Gurdjieff
Beelzebub's Tales to his Grandson, Book III
Routledge and Keegan Paul 1974

PRESENT

We glimpse the past darkly through our emotions.
We glimpse the future brightly through our emotions.
We rarely glimpse the present at all!

We can only evolve if we achieve the wisdom to keep the past in balance with the future.
If we fail to do this, we will lose our identity as a genus species.
This is a baby in the bathwater!
This is not something we throw away!

The present is the thread that connects us to who we were and who we are going to be.
Wisdom dictates we should not repeat the mistakes of the past.
Awareness dictates we should not be prisoners of distortion.
Understanding dictates that we should not live in the future.
This truth is the baby in the bathwater!
This is not something we should throw away!

If we do not understand that we should live in the present, then we will distort both the past and the future.

"Now there are three steps to heaven,
Just listen and you will plainly see.
And as I travel on,
And things do go wrong,
Just call it steps one, two and three."

Bob and Eddie Cochran
Three Steps to Heaven, 1960

PROCESS

Distortion can occur in our minds, our spirit,
our bodies or our emotions or our language.
Such change will manifest on all levels of our being.
This process can be seen in the same form whether triggered
by internal causes, psychological events or external situations.
We make no distinction about trauma from any source.
Our response will be disease and death or healing and growth.
The wave-like reaction to trauma reflects through the mirror.
The wave-like response to contentment also reflects through the mirror.
Thus we react in equal and opposite forms to the impact of change.
Thus we respond in exact manner, reversed through the mirror.
Over time, we begin to understand.
With experience, we become aware.
With awareness, we achieve knowledge.
With knowledge, we discover wisdom.
With wisdom, we learn kindness.
With kindness, we abandon the hierarchy.

"But what happened to the poor fox? Long after, the prince went once
again into the wood, and there met the fox, who said, "You have now
everything that you can desire, but to my misfortune there is no end,
although it lies in your power to release me." And with tears, it begged
the prince to cut off its head and feet. At last the prince did so; and
scarcely was it accomplished when the fox became a man, who was no
other that the brother of the princess, delivered at length from the charm
which bound him."

The Golden Bird
Fairy Tales from Grimm
Wells Gardner Darton and Co 1948

SCAPEGOAT

We do not understand the Other.
They threaten us with their difference and their similarity.
In order to perceive the Other,
we have to separate ourselves away from them.
Trauma is the usual tool!
This act is the cornerstone of the hierarchy.
Distortion of our awareness is the result and the cause of it.
Once we are separate from the Other,
we can project our fear onto them to relieve our own pain.
Thus we administer pain to Others.
Also, reversed through the Mirror, we reflect our own pain to inflict guilt.
Which stance we take depends upon our perception of events
and the permission we allow ourselves and Others.
Which stance we take depends upon the language we use,
the dance we are dancing and the song we are singing.
For as long as we give ourselves permission,
we can glare at the Other to forgive ourselves.
For as long as we are diseased,
we can blame the Other to explain our distorted reflection.
It's them, not me!
For as long as we are in pain, we will need someone to blame.
Why have allowed ourselves permission to come to this pass?

"Have you seen the old girl who walks the streets of London,
Dirt in her hair and her clothes in rags?
She's no time for talking, she just keeps on walking,
Carrying her home in two carrier bags."

Ralph McTell
The Streets of London, 1968

SINGING

Once we understand how to give ourselves permission
to use our own language, we can begin to sing our own song.
This is our song of destiny.

Once we can sing, we can circle and spiral around Others.
Friend or enemy?
Love or hate?
Life or death?
We can sing a hierarchy into existence
to separate ourselves from the universe.
We can talk the language of past and language of future.
We can talk language of defeat or language of wisdom.
As if they meant anything!
We can talk about what we want, what we don't want,
what we need, what we don't need.
We can look at everything through the mirror.
We can use our palate to make fine equations.
What do we hear from our singing?
Can we bring it into harmony?
Can we understand?
Can we find contentment?
Is there harmony in the spheres?

"I've taken my bows
And my curtain calls.
You brought me fame and fortune
And everything that goes with it,
But it's been no bed of roses, no pleasure cruise;
I consider it a challenge before the whole human race,
And I ain't gonna lose."

Freddie Mercury and Queen
We Are The Champions, 1977

SPIRAL

To avoid weak and distorted thinking,
it is important to use all our palate of knowledge
to gather all possible information into a circle of illumination.
Our equations should consider the stream of consciousness.
Each circle forms part of a spiral of existence.
These spirals spin the magnetic and electric energy
that creates the universe.
Dancing and singing, we trace out our footsteps
through our environment as we study our reflected image in the mirror.
This process is triggered by any movement, by any stasis.
This process will occur despite us, without us, within us.
We circle round and round.
We travel on spiral pathways.
We discover our direction.
We manoeuvre around existence.
With each new fact, truth changes.
With each new turn, experience grows.
With each new turn, awareness is gained.
With each new turn, we evolve.
Confusion is a healthy state.
Its presence proves our feet upon the path.
Permission to proceed with wisdom is all we need.

"You're the kind of person you meet at certain dismal, dull affairs,
Centre of a crowd, talking much too loud,
Running up and down the stairs.
It seems to me that you have seen too much in too few years,
And though you try, you can't hide;
Your eyes are edged with tears."

Mick Jagger and Keith Richards
Nineteenth Nervous Breakdown, 1965

STRENGTH

In order to become strong, we must grow and thrive.
We have to heal from disease and trauma and find balance.
We need a full palate of knowledge, and the experience to use it wisely. In
order to achieve strength, we have to know who we are,
what we have been and what we can become.
We have to be honest enough to come to grips with our own true nature.
To be honest, humans make Tyrannosaurus Rex look like puppy dogs!
In order to test our strength, we need to pit this strength
against something to see how mortal or immortal we actually are!
If we direct it at Others, we cause trauma,
which comes around and goes around until we experience it as fate.
This locks us into a closed circle,
which cannot take us to the open spiral of the universe.
Instead, we go round and round in disease and distortion
until our orbit collapses and we start to spin the other way.
Healthy life spins in a centrifugal manner,
allowing for growth and evolution.
If we collapse in on ourselves, we change our shape,
we reverse through the mirror and we begin to die.
It would be far better to perceive the true enemy
(our own fragmented psyche) and to finally know our true friend
(the universe is our natural home and we have family here).
We can allow awareness and evolve to the point when we can begin to
perceive the nature of existence and find our true place within it,
rather than just tearing up the place because we are in pain of our own making.
Consciousness is painfully wrought from our species, but it is in our
potential to achieve this if we give ourselves the permission to do it.

"These late eclipses in the sun and moon portend no good to us. Though
the wisdom of nature can reason it thus and thus, yet nature finds itself
scourged by the subsequent effects. Love cools, mutinies; in countries
discord; in palaces treason; and the bond cracked between son and father."

King Lear
William Shakespeare

TRUTH

With every new fact, truth changes.
Truth is a moveable feast.
What is true now may not have been true in the past,
or remain true in the future.
Truth moves its goalposts depending on when and where we are,
what we know, what we discover later.
A new discovery or understanding changes truth.

We used to know but now we're not so sure!

Truth has often meant different things to different people.
Has it ever meant the same thing to all of us?
Throughout existence we have made a friend of our enemy
and an enemy of our friend.
We have known before what we discover tomorrow,
but our language changes, so our perceptions change.
We knew things before we had language to study and observe.
The truth is that the universe is fulfilling its potential, but are we?
The truth is that life and death are reflections in the mirror.
The truth is that love will always enable life and death.
The truth is that hate will always enable disease and healing.
The truth is that we can learn to do this consciously.
The truth is that we only need to give ourselves permission to understand.

"The deep within the deep,
The superior man is a teacher
And practices what he preaches.
Because of his sincerity
He is said the have a penetrating mind."

Sam Reifler
I Ching, Hexagram 29
Bantam 1981

UNDERSTAND

We started with only appetite to satisfy.
We survived for aeons without thinking about it, without language.
We evolved thinking and language to exploit niches in the environment,
niches that enabled us to become dominant in a hostile universe.
This is where we grew strong and proliferated.

We have forgotten this past.
We faced the present then, but we can't see it now.
We faced the future when we planted grain and domesticated animals.
What future do we see now?
We knew the future when we forged our trade routes
and developed religion.
We planned for the future when we forged iron and conquered Others.
We fear the future as we build our bombs to destroy our enemy.
We fear the past, because it shows us
who we really are and what we are capable of.
We have forgotten the present.
We ignore our potential for life if we indulge our fear of death.
We are disease.
We poison the environment and rape the universe.
We are acting as death!
We are in a downward spiral.
We are slaves to our appetites and our fears.
We drive Others before us ragged and dying as we satisfy our own needs.
We have forgotten the future.

"Living is easy with eyes closed,
Misunderstanding all you see.
It's getting hard to be someone, but it all works out.
It doesn't matter much to me."

John Lennon and Paul McCartney
Strawberry Fields Forever, 1967

UNIVERSE

The universe is beyond our knowledge.
Survival in the environment has always been difficult,
but we have always been here.
The past bears witness to our record, but the future may forget us.
All we ever have is the present.
We have no guarantee of survival.
Our motivation must allow us to try for life.
Our manoeuvres must allow us a chance for life.
Our permission must include our potential for life.
Dancing and singing, we circle and spiral,
round and round in the stream of consciousness.

There are only two signposts in hell.
One way says, this feels okay. The other one says, this doesn't.

If we dance towards distortion and disease, we will find death.
If we dance towards healing and contentment, we will find life.
If we dance in the footsteps of our ancestors, we can explore our environment.
But we must forge our own dance steps if we are to evolve.
We can sing the songs of our ancestors,
but we must sing our own song if we are to find our destiny.
We must dance our own dance, sing our own song.
If we embrace life, all the dances and songs will become the universe.
If we embrace death, the universe will become more and more different
and discordant until everything ceases.

"Not of mother, nor of father was my creation
I was made from the ninefold elements
From fruit trees, from paradisal fruit;
From primroses and hillflowers, from the blossom of the trees and bushes;
From the roots of the earth I was made; from the water of the ninth wave."

John Matthews
Taliesin Cad Goddeu
Aquarian 1991

WISDOM

Why do mystics allude to bees?
They have been used as mystic symbols for aeons.

It is obvious that as we become individually conscious,
we will see the Others all around us as we perceive the hive.
We do not immediately recognise our kinship as we fight for freedom.

In fear, we are alone, even though we are surrounded by life.

We continue this illusion by hiding in the hierarchy
to separate us from Others, invoking fate.
Our actions are exactly mirrored by the universe,
and so we create our destiny.

Dancing away from life ensures magnetic discharge.
The discharge pattern will be an exact reflection of the original act.
Electric energy discharges as a consequence of this action.

Singing our song of independence,
the melody reflected back is the distortion we cause.

For every action there is an equal and opposite reaction.

By their footsteps thou shalt know them.

"Come on guys, cheer up.
Worse things happen at sea, you know.
I mean, what have you got to lose?
You know, you came from nothing,
You're going back to nothing.
What have you lost? Nothing!"

Eric Idle
Always Look on the Bright Side of Life, 1979

www.ingramcontent.com/pod-product-compliance
Lightning Source LLC
Chambersburg PA
CBHW020433290526
45785CB00002B/834